Praise for *Breaking the Barnyard Barrier*

"Hats off to Linda Rhodes for her masterful storytelling as a veterinarian, innovator, and entrepreneur. *Breaking the Barnyard Barrier* is a wildly entertaining and inspiring ride through life's defining moments shaped by curiosity, courage, and a steadfast moral compass—a true testament to what's possible!"

—Kristin Peck, CEO, Zoetis

"I thoroughly enjoyed reading *Breaking the Barnyard Barrier*, the parallel personal and professional stories, the story of our lives as vets. The family life and background were so interesting and inspiring. As the book describes—life is what you make it, a deeply emotional journey, making hard choices and moving on and taking it all in—the landscapes and the relationships. The story is told beautifully, laying it open sometimes in raw and deeply personal reflections, and with humility and grace among the triumphs, trials, and tribulations."

—Andrew Hoffman, Gilbert S. Kahn Dean, School of Veterinary Medicine, University of Pennsylvania

"*Breaking the Barnyard Barrier* is a stunning memoir by Linda Rhodes, who takes readers on a journey from her student days to the truly climactic scenes of birthing cows in the male bastion of Utah's dairy farms. Despite doors closed to her postgraduation, and then through the challenges of young marriage, this wonderful veterinarian definitely (and defiantly) is honest to a fault. Revealing the many affronts faced, Rhodes shares how she practiced medicine with dignity and the kindest of hearts—the sort that all females in labor appreciate and remember forever."

—Marcia Bradley, author of *The Home for Wayward Girls*, instructor at Sarah Lawrence College

"Dr. Rhodes does an incredible job taking the reader along her journey to achieving her dream of becoming a large animal veterinarian at a time when such a thing—a lady cow vet—really didn't exist! You get to ride shotgun with Dr. Rhodes as she navigates the challenges and prejudices and her personal struggles on her way to fulfilling her life's dream. The story is well written and enjoyable, although sometimes frustrating to read as you learn of all the obstacles Dr. Rhodes had to overcome. If you have ever wondered what it takes to be a veterinarian, much less a woman veterinarian in a man's world, and to come out on top, this is a must read!"

—Douglas Mader, author of *The Vet at Noah's Ark: Stories of Survival from an Inner City Animal Hospital*

BREAKING THE BARNYARD BARRIER

Breaking the Barnyard Barrier

A Woman Veterinarian Paves the Way

LINDA RHODES

UNIVERSITY OF NEVADA PRESS | *Reno & Las Vegas*

University of Nevada Press | Reno, Nevada 89557 USA
www.unpress.nevada.edu
Copyright © 2026 by University of Nevada Press
Photographs © 2026 by Linda Rhodes

Manufactured in the United States of America

FIRST PRINTING

Cover design by Diane McIntosh

Library of Congress Cataloging-in-Publication Data is on file.

ISBN 978-1-64779-235-0 (paper)
ISBN 978-1-64779-236-7 (ebook)
LCCN: 2025029899

The paper used in this book meets the requirements of
American National Standard for Information Sciences—
Permanence of Paper for Printed Library Materials,
ANSI/NISO Z39.48-1992 (R2002).

To my son, Adam

Contents

BREAKING THE BARNYARD BARRIER

Prologue
C-Section in Utah

I SANK ONTO THE DECREPIT red couch exhausted after a long day of shuttling from cow barn to sheep shed in the bitter November cold of Logan, Utah. The moonlight was so bright it threw shadows in the field, the only sound a gentle breeze rustling the pine trees. My husband, Vincent, was perched on a stool near the woodstove, putting a new set of strings on his old flat-topped guitar. The *Salt Lake Tribune* was folded next to me, with an article about the Camp David Peace Accords and something about Jimmy Carter I was too tired to read. My cat Logan was asleep on the rag rug.

The old black rotary phone gave a loud, sharp, elongated ring, cutting the silence, making Logan stand straight up, tail twitching. I jumped to grab it before the second ring.

"Dr. Rhodes here," I said, trying out a deeper voice to sound professional. I was getting used to the fact that I finally was a real doctor now, although I didn't often feel like it. After my first few months of starting my work in large animal medicine at Utah State University, the general hubbub about having a woman as the new intern had died down.

"Dr. Rhodes, this is Spencer, from the dairy." Spencer was the backup dairy manager, working nights. "Gotta situation here— calving trouble." He sounded out of breath.

"What's the problem?" I asked. This was my first calving call, and my heart started beating faster. Spencer and the cowboys at the barn could handle routine calvings. For him to call me meant this one was going to be a challenge.

"Only got one foot out, she's been pushing awhile, no progress." *Awhile* meant the guys at the barn had been trying for hours to pull that calf with no success. Something was seriously wrong. A tough calving, my first on my own. What-ifs starting rattling around in my head. What if I couldn't figure out the calf's position? What if I wasn't strong enough to pull it? What if it was twins, or dead, or backward?

I took a deep breath.

"Be there soon," I said. Vincent looked up, frowned, and set his guitar down.

"You going on a call?" he asked. It was pretty obvious. I nodded.

"Okay, I'm headed to bed soon." He picked up the guitar and strummed a blues chord. "See you in the morning."

I grabbed clean coveralls, scooped up the truck keys, and shrugged into my coat. My truck was chilly. The heater kicked in at the end of the long dirt driveway. I could see down into the valley, the spire of the Temple lit with moonlight. The dairy was a short drive from my house, and I had ten minutes of increasing worry as I imagined all the things that might go wrong, and how awkward it would be if I couldn't handle it and had to call for help from my boss, a much more experienced vet. The staff at the Department of Animal, Dairy, and Veterinary Science consisted entirely of men, and I was sure they were waiting for me to fail, which would confirm the fact that a woman's place was in the home, washing their coveralls and cooking their meals.

I pulled up to the Utah State University dairy barn and switched off the truck. The familiar smell of cow manure and silage hit me as I went around the back to get my kit. I found Spencer and a couple of cowhands standing around a big Holstein with one large, black-and-white calf hoof sticking out of her vagina. Spencer and his crew were responsible for the evening milking of the two hundred or so cows, hosing down the milking parlor afterward, and then around nine p.m. doing the night walkthrough, including checking on the cows in the calving area of the barn. He was no taller than me, stocky and muscular, a shock of blond hair sticking out of his baseball cap. The three young cowhands looked remarkably similar—tall, fair, blue jeans, men with large capable hands and strong backs. They likely grew up around cows and had more experience than I did pulling calves. They had moved this poor cow into a well-lit area with a deep sink. I noticed bloody calving chains on the floor. Calving chains are a fixture in dairy barns—five-foot-long stainless steel chains that can be looped around a calf's feet to apply traction and slide it out of the vaginal canal. If the chains were out, it meant they'd been trying to pull the calf for too long before calling me. Likely they felt calling the vet intern was the last resort.

Silent, they all stared at the floor, not meeting my gaze. I felt bad for the cow, her head hanging down, breathing hard, her vulva bruised and swollen. I laid a hand on her warm flank to give myself a moment to think and watched her belly contract with another push. Poor girl, she must be exhausted.

My skills at helping a cow to calve were rudimentary. At University of Pennsylvania Veterinary School, I had learned a great deal about various procedures for repositioning a calf to ease a delivery. But the calvings in which I had assisted were routine, a minor adjustment of a leg, or a bit of pulling, but this wasn't going to be easy. This calf was stuck.

I lubed up my plastic sleeve and reached in to work out the calf's position. The big foot was wedged in the cow's vaginal canal. Where was the other foot? It must be farther forward in the uterus than I could reach. The leg twitched when I pinched it, so at least the calf was alive. This stressed calf had been through a rough time the past few hours, I suspected, with cowhands with their large muscular arms trying to push or pull the poor thing. Brute force wouldn't solve this problem, and even my slender arm couldn't ease far enough in the vaginal canal to determine how to proceed. Spencer was standing next to me, holding the cow's tail, eager to help somehow. The other guys were leaning against the wall, watching me, each chewing on a stalk of hay, expressions neutral. Mormon cowboys didn't chew tobacco. I had a fleeting thought that they had probably never seen a women veterinarian at work, and I couldn't tell if they were amused or annoyed.

Perhaps more lube and repositioning could get this calf out, or maybe a C-section was needed. The size of the foot—that was my key. That damn foot was huge. A vaginal delivery was unlikely.

"Bull calf," Spencer said. The cowboys nodded solemnly. Given the size of the foot they were probably right. This little bull, all hundred and fifty pounds of him, by the look of his foot, would normally have squirted right out of his mom, flapped his wet ears and been up and bawling in ten minutes. Now he was stuck. I hoped he hadn't given up.

"Back foot?" Spencer asked. A normal calving is two front feet and the nose first. In my reproduction course, I scored an Excellent and had memorized hundreds of procedures but seeing the drawing on the page was nothing like standing in a cold barn with a calf's foot in my face. I was going to figure this out, I told myself, despite my lack of experience and the knot in my gut. I rolled my shoulders back and took a deep breath.

A veterinary school lecture on reproduction played out in my head.

Start at the foot, run your hand down the leg, feel as far as possible in the cow's vaginal canal. You will run into either the tail or the nose.

I stood on my tiptoes and stretched, my chest pressed to the rear of the cow, my arm up to the armpit in her vagina, running my hand along the calf's impossibly long leg. The cow bellowed, the tortured sound echoing in the barn. *Sorry, girl*, I thought.

"Okay, I've got the tail, it's a hind leg," I said. Progress! I was figuring this out. It was only six months ago that I was clutching my diploma in West Philadelphia, dreaming of being in the dairy barn. And here I was, with the first difficult calving of my career.

While I groped around, the cow's contractions squeezed my arm, making my hand nearly numb. I would have to be the one not only to declare that a C-section was needed but also to do it. I knew it was my call. I had a momentary urge to run back to my house, get my surgery textbook and bone up on C-sections. I glanced over at the straw chewers, leaning against the wall, hands in their pockets. They were calmly staring, waiting for me to perform some magic and slide the calf out so they could go home and eat the late supper their wives were probably keeping warm in the oven. A C-section would mean at least another couple of hours in the barn. And Spencer most likely thought the veterinarian should be able to pull a stuck calf. He would be sure to spread the story around if this didn't go well. Ending up with a dead calf—or worse, a dead calf and a dead cow—would be a hard hole to dig myself out of in a world where I was the first woman vet any of these men had seen.

"Okay, guys," I said, with more confidence than I felt, "I think this is a C-section."

"Come on, you're kidding. You can't straighten that calf and pull it?" Spencer said, annoyed. One of the cowboys pulled his cap off and dusted his leg with it, frowning.

"The calf is breech, there's no way to get that second back leg into position," I said, trying to sound sure of it. These fellows would have to get with the program, because at this point, there was no choice. I was making the call and needed their help.

"Yup, C-section. Let's get her cleaned up," I said. "You guys get me a couple of buckets of hot water." Once I decided, I was sure. *The girl vet is going to do surgery you guys*, I thought to myself. *Surprise, surprise.*

"Spencer, get the clippers, we need to get the hair off her left side where I'll make the incision."

Spencer, his mouth an angry line, was not used to a woman giving orders. He went to fetch the clippers and an extension cord. I walked outside. The night was black, the only light from a few stars sparkling in the cold mountain air fragrant with pine and sage. The moon was setting behind the black mass of the mountain range. I took a deep breath and leaned against the cold metal of my truck. God, it had been a long road to this barn, this night, this responsibility. So many times, I could have turned back. I was told it was too hard, women couldn't do this work, I should try something easier.

Yet, here I was, in this barn in the middle of this dark, silent night in Utah, and it was time to do my first C-section. It was terrifying, but I knew I could do it.

Think, Linda, think. *Incision on the left side because it's easier to work around the rumen than the small intestines on the right side. Okay, okay, that's right. That's good. Lift the uterus up to the incision and hold it to prevent contamination of the abdominal cavity. Make the uterine incision, remove the calf.* The mental rehearsal helped, although my heart beat fast and hard. I could hear banging back in the barn—they were starting to wonder where I was. *Uterine incision, grab the calf, pull it out, stitch up.*

Spencer was hard at work shaving the thick black hair from the left side of the cow, clippers buzzing. The cow strained hard, groaning. She had been in labor way too long, poor thing, and I knew she was getting weaker.

"She's just about tuckered out," Spencer said. I nodded. He did care about his cows.

Epidural! The word suddenly appeared in my head. I needed to give her an epidural so she wouldn't strain during the surgery. Good, I was remembering. I stuck a needle between her last couple of vertebrae and the yellow-tinged cerebrospinal fluid flowed into the syringe as I pulled back on the plunger. Perfect. I willed the cow not to move so I could infuse the lidocaine. Spencer and the cowboys were standing behind me, silently, eyes boring into my head. I had an itchy feeling they were waiting for the girl vet to do something stupid. But in fact, the lidocaine was working. The poor old cow stopped straining and grunting, and her tail went limp. Even the cowboys could see that was a good start. *Don't worry, old girl,* I thought. *I'm gonna help you.*

I would have to do my best to keep things clean. Sterile was impossible in the barn. A cesarean section in a cow is done standing—that is, the cow is standing, her head in a rope halter tied to something sturdy. The uterus can be accessed from either her right or left side. The surgeon faces the selected side of the cow and makes the incision high on the flank, starting in front of the point of the hip and angling forward. The incision should be about sixteen inches long.

Two large syringes of lidocaine injected along my planned incision line on the upper left side of the cow numbed her so she wouldn't feel pain during the procedure. I scrubbed my hands in the deep sink with antiseptic soap bright orange with iodine. The barn was quiet now. The cow had stopped moaning and grunting, and the guys were uncomfortable with small talk. It was coming up on midnight. The scrubbing calmed me down. Iodine stung where my cuticles were chewed raw, a bad habit begun during the stress of vet school.

"Okay, gentlemen, let's get started," I said.

I snapped the large scalpel blade onto the handle. The barn got even quieter. I took a deep breath. I was now in my world; this was my surgery. The incision felt right—a smooth, sure cut, followed by small beads of blood, deep through the tough leather skin and into the muscular layers on the side of the abdomen. The lidocaine was doing its job—the cow didn't flinch. I deepened the cut. A small artery severed by the incision spurted bright red, speckling my glasses. I tied it off and cut into the abdomen.

After a clean cut through the muscles, the gleaming pink uterus bulged up through the incision. I reached into the cow's belly and ran my hand along its smooth curve until I stood on tiptoe to feel the bottom edge. It was as big as a fifty-five-gallon drum. How the hell was I going to lift the uterus up far enough to keep all the amniotic fluid from dumping into the abdominal cavity? With the calf inside, it weighed at least two hundred pounds. Damn it, this was going to be a mess. I felt the calf shift inside. He was big, he was stressed, and I knew I had to get him out quickly. I sent a mental message to the calf: *Help is coming.*

I backed out of the cow's belly, my hands dripping in blood and mucus, coveralls soaked through and took a deep breath. By now, the sterile field was contaminated with barn dust and worse, but I tried to use sterile technique anyway. Plunging my arm back in, I heaved the uterus up toward the incision as best I could with my left hand while using my right hand to make a clean eighteen-inch cut. Thick amniotic fluid, smelling slightly sweet, sloshed everywhere. I reached my right arm into the uterus and felt the jumble of legs, torso, head, tail.

It's gonna be alright, big boy. Hold on a few more minutes, I thought. I didn't dare say this out loud, for fear the cowboys would mock me.

"Get the chains, Spencer!" I yelled. He snatched a set of calving chains, metal clattering as he ran over, while I grabbed a leg. My breath was shallow, my heart pounding in my chest. Time sped up. Every second counted. The calf needed to get some air into his lungs if he was going to survive.

"I'll hold the feet, you loop the chains on them, then you guys lift!"

The barn was suddenly noisy with the chains rattling, the cow bellowing again. Spencer looped a chain around the foot I was clutching while I groped around feeling for the other leg. I seized the first leg I found and held up the hoof for Spencer.

The guys grabbed the chains and heaved the calf upward, grunting and pulling. But that damn calf didn't budge. I realized, in my haste, I hadn't checked the legs. Spencer and crew were pulling on one front leg and one hind leg, and there was no way a 150-pound calf was going to come through that incision sideways.

"Wait, loosen up. Take that chain off!" I yelled. One of the cowboys hanging on to the hind foot unwrapped the chain and let it go. I shoved my arm back into the uterus and found the second front foot.

"This one—pull on this one!"

I reached for the calf's head and straightened out the neck that was twisted backward. My thumb slipped into the calf's mouth, and he gave a suck, as if my thumb was his mother's teat. A rush of gratitude flowed over me—he was alive! With a tremendous yank, Spencer and his helper had the little guy out on the barn floor, coughing and sputtering, gasping for breath. What a messy process this was, and yet here was a perfectly formed bull calf covered in slippery mucus, hair wet through, floppy little ears, all black like his mother except for white patches on his legs. Spencer and the cowboys grinned at one another. We all felt this miracle of birth, chaotic and hectic as it was.

"Get him upside down," I commanded. They each grabbed a hind leg and held him as high as they could, head down. At least a gallon of mucus drained out his nose, splashing on the barn floor. He took a tremendous breath and shook his head, wet ears flapping.

"He's breathing!" Spencer exclaimed. "Biggest dang bull calf I've seen in a long time."

I grinned. My first C-section. I made the call, I did the surgery, and both the mother and calf were going to make it. I felt like hugging them both, and the cowboys too. I turned away so Spencer wouldn't see my tears of relief. It wouldn't do for the rumor to get out that the vet cried when she delivered the calf.

Plus, I was too busy to celebrate. The mother needed my help now. "The little guy will be fine. Get some towels and dry him off so he doesn't get cold," I said, still clutching the sides of the uterine incision. We were a mess—bloody, wet, slimy. Spencer whistled as he dried off the calf and the cowboys got busy mopping up. Maybe they would grudgingly admit that, in fact, that girl intern did okay, even if she did look awful in her soaked coveralls with her face spattered with blood.

The mama cow turned her neck toward her son and lowed softly. So lovely to hear that maternal greeting to her newborn. By now it was after one a.m., but I was full of energy. I could be exhausted later. Now, I still had a lot of stitching to do. The cow and calf would have died if I hadn't had the knowledge of surgery and the courage to do it. This is what I trained for, all those long years of veterinary school. Something so concrete and real, my contribution, my purpose. I could put up with the doubters, the scoffers, the rudeness, as long as I could look at a poor old mother cow and know that I helped her through a difficult night.

A truck door slammed outside.

"My heck," Spencer exclaimed. "Who could be coming by this late?"

Dr. Nelson stuck his head in the door. "Everything okay in here?" he said, looking at the mess, smiling at the newborn. My boss, in the middle of the night. One of the cowboys had probably called him to say the new intern was attempting a C-section. I imagined him in bed, tossing and turning next to his wife, wondering if I could pull it off, until he couldn't stand it anymore and had to come check on me.

Dr. Lamar Nelson was a Utah native, a blond-haired, blue-eyed churchgoing Mormon, a tenured faculty member at Utah State University. A tall, straight-backed man in his mid-fifties, his coveralls clean, his rubber boots scrubbed, hair combed back from his forehead.

"Looks like you've got everything under control," he said as he gazed across the pile of dirty surgical instruments on the card table, to the gaping incision in the cow, to me, still holding the sides of the uterus, my coveralls soaked to my armpits, my face and glasses speckled with blood.

"Want a hand stitching up?" Dr. Nelson offered.

"Sure, Dr. Nelson, thanks. There's another pair of gloves in my truck."

I was glowing with pride that I had pulled off the C-section. Thank God Dr. Nelson wasn't here when I'd tried to pull the calf out sidewise. We stood side by side, Dr. Nelson holding up the uterus while I stitched, tying off sutures and being sure to invert the edges for a good seal. I waited for him to tell me what a good job I had done, how it was all quite impressive for a new graduate, but I guess it didn't occur to him that I might need reassurance.

The layers of muscle came together nicely, and finally skin, each stitch carefully pulled to the right tension. He leaned on the cow's side and cut the stitches as I placed them.

What about the placenta? I hadn't cut the umbilical cord. It must have ruptured when the guys lifted the calf out. I decided not to mention it. I'd look it up when I got home.

"You sure do a neat stitching job. I guess that's a girl thing," he said. I glanced over—was he kidding? A flash of anger washed over me. *A girl thing?* Damn it. This wasn't embroidery. This wasn't just me trying to prove I could handle the work. I was pioneering for all women who might want to practice large animal medicine. If I failed, then these cowboys would use that, however unfairly, as evidence that women just weren't cut out for the job.

My anger faded into exhaustion as I tied the last skin suture and tugged my gloves off. Dr. Nelson had tried to give me a compliment about my surgical technique, and I decided to take it.

Spencer piled the towels in a heap and finished mopping the bloody floor.

"Doc," Spencer said, "I'm gonna head home. That okay?"

"Sure," Dr. Nelson and I both said simultaneously.

I realized I was not "Doc" to Spencer. Not yet.

Dr. Nelson patted the cow's rump. "Okay, Spencer, just get this old girl back in the hospital pen first."

Getting the calf's legs mixed up wasn't such a big mistake, I told myself. And without my decision to even do the surgery, that calf would be dead by now—and probably his mama too. I'll get there, I told myself. Someday.

"You okay?" Dr. Nelson asked, pulling off his surgical gloves. "That was some heavy sigh."

"Just tired," I said. It would take a lot more than one C-section for the Utah cowhands to consider me a real Doc. But I had proved that I had enough guts and knowledge to save this calf and his mother, and that was a wondrous thing. I had applied my book learning, conquered my fear, and done the job, even if it wasn't terribly elegant. I took a deep breath and felt my heart expand with pride.

❖

Showered, hair damp, I slid into bed next to Vincent, who was fast asleep. The sun would be up in an hour. The house was chilly. Warm waves of the waterbed rocked me gently, but I couldn't sleep. My first C-section. It wasn't as polished as I would have liked, but not bad for a beginner. I better go back this morning and give the cow antibiotics. All that contaminated amniotic fluid in her abdomen. Damn—should have done it last night. My eyes got heavy. I stretched my toes into the warm waterbed and slept.

Peach and pink wispy clouds drifted over the mountains at dawn. I drove back to the dairy, past undulating fallow fields of alfalfa, Black Angus cows grazing on the grass glistening with the overnight frost. The first light glowed on the steeple of the Logan Temple. Cache Valley was framed with the jagged peaks of the snow-dusted Wasatch Mountains.

With fresh coveralls and clean boots, I gulped hot coffee from my thermos. The milkers had started the day, and the whirring sound of the milking machines echoed in the barn. My patient was standing in the hospital stall, swooshing her tail, and munching alfalfa hay. Her suture line was a bit swollen, but no sign of discharge or infection, at least not yet. Amazing what cows can tolerate. I leaned my arms on the wooden stall and sighed, pleased with my work. The coffee was no use, I was ready to crawl up in the haymow and sleep for a couple of hours. Instead, I went to the truck and got a bottle of penicillin—she needed a dose of antibiotics.

No one else was at the office this early. I typed up my case report, left it on Dr. Nelson's desk, and went home to sleep. I returned after lunchtime and ran into Clem Marten, the extension veterinarian, in the hall. Extension veterinarians were employed by state universities, for the purpose of extending the learning from the university to the farm community. They were supposed to translate the university's research on nutrition, calf health, and manure disposal for dairy farms to help Utah farmers figure out how best to put the academic research to use. Clem was a beef cattle specialist. He stood straight as a lodgepole pine, dark shiny hair, clear brown eyes, cowboy hat in hand. He hadn't tipped his hand about what he thought of a woman intern. Polite, remote, and just friendly enough, Clem was someone I hadn't figured out yet.

"Heard you did a C-section last night." Just a statement of fact, with a slight smile. I didn't expect a "Good for you" from Clem.

Yes, I'll bet he did hear, and everyone else in the department too. Surely this was the first time in the history of Utah State University dairy that a woman had done a C-section. They should be impressed, but I was pretty sure the reaction wouldn't be all positive. It didn't completely challenge their worldview of what a woman should be doing, but it shook it up enough to be uncomfortable.

"Your first?" he said. He smiled and tilted his head. Maybe this was going to be a compliment after all.

"Yes," I shrugged.

"Live bull calf," he stated. He had heard the story. "And you did it standing, from the left?"

"Yup."

"We don't generally do it that way out here," he said in a neutral kind of voice.

You don't? Now are you going to tell me exactly what I did wrong? The cow is doing fine, the calf is doing fine, what the hell is wrong with my way? I gulped back my annoyance.

"How do you do it?" I put on my most pleasant *well isn't that nice* kind of voice.

"We go in from the right," Clem said.

I recalled reading in my reproduction textbook that morning.

"If the approach is from the right, and the incision is extended a bit too ventrally, it is difficult to hold the intestines within the abdomen. If the cow strains, coughs, or struggles, an armful of intestines may be expelled through the laparotomy incision and occasionally the cow may put her foot through them."

I liked my way better.

PART ONE

Barriers

CHAPTER 1

I EMERGED FROM THE CRAMPED car, stretched my arms over my head, and took a deep breath. The sweet scent of lilacs was a wonderful change from the stench of West Philadelphia. My sister, Anne, carried her daughter, Satya, seven years old, fast asleep, into the house. Vincent pulled boxes out of the car and piled them on the driveway. The chickens ran to greet us, cackling, looking for their dinner of corn. The setting sun cast a warm light on the meadow, and the peepers sang down by the pond. Vincent put his arm around me. We stood, silent, and gazed at the rolling green hills east of the house. I leaned my head on his shoulder.

Vincent sighed.

"What?" I asked.

"Long day," he said.

After my Philadelphia life was packed up and the rental cleaned so I could get my deposit back, we left Philly around three in the afternoon, arriving in Freeville, New York, a few miles outside of Ithaca, after four hours on the road. Anne, Satya, and Vincent came to Philadelphia to celebrate my graduation from Penn Veterinary School in late May 1978. I had just turned twenty-nine, and after four years of living apart from him, I was ready to start my life with Vincent—and, hopefully, a job as a large animal veterinarian in the rolling hills and meadows around Ithaca, New York.

❖

Anne, Vincent, and a group of musicians and friends lived communally in an old Victorian house in Freeville while I was studying in Philadelphia. Now I was happily done with living in a city and the rigors of veterinary school. We had planned to settle into a life—Vincent playing music with his brothers, me working as a large animal vet in the local dairy farms. It would be so good if we could finally be together after four years of Vincent in Freeville and me living in the gritty world of West Philadelphia, but in spite of months of trying, I hadn't found a job. We both knew that meant our dream was in jeopardy, but we avoided talking about what might come next.

For now, it was enough to breathe the scent of lilacs and lean on each other. The screen door banged. Anne threw some cracked corn out the back door for the chickens, already busy pecking. I plopped down on the porch steps.

"Seems weird not to have a schedule," I said. My life had been defined for the last four years by a hectic rush of classes, labs, and clinics.

Vincent smiled. "Maybe you can take a few weeks to slow down," he said.

My back against the porch railing, I stretched my legs out. The peepers down by the pond were getting louder, fireflies flashed in the grass, the last of the light slanted across the meadow.

"I guess I could try that," I said, and we both laughed.

"It's getting dark," Vincent said. "I'll get your stuff and put it in the cabin."

The Freeville house functioned as a commune, with most of the original founders who had moved into the house in 1974, when I moved to Philly, still there. During the four years I toiled away at vet school, the vegetable garden had grown large and weedy, a few more cats had turned up, and the attic and basement filled with the boxes and miscellaneous detritus of various musicians who came and went.

The cabin, a tiny one-room shed behind the house, would be fine for now, but I hoped in a few weeks I would find a job with a salary so that Vincent and I could move someplace to avoid the chaos of the commune. I wanted to celebrate finally being Dr. Rhodes, but instead I worried. Starting in early spring of 1978, long before graduation, I searched for a job in large animal practice, but it had gradually become clear that finding a job taking care of cows near Freeville was going to be much harder than I had expected. Degree in hand, no job, student loan payments due in a couple of months, I had a bank account so close to zero that the bank might close it out.

The countryside around Freeville was filled with dairy farms. New York State was the third largest producer of milk, after Wisconsin and California. Prosperous dairy farms dotted the landscape. Since the beginning of vet school, my plan had been to return to Freeville. I'd spent the spring of my senior year interviewing for all the jobs listed in the area. No one would hire me.

The pink sunset clouds darkened to gray. Anne was in the kitchen singing along with the radio. She chopped zucchini and onions into the oil-coated wok, making stir-fry for dinner. The light was on in Vincent's little cabin. I rolled my shoulders, stretched to reach my toes, and yawned. My exhaustion from the last four years settled over me like a heavy blanket. There was still a long way to go until I was a practicing veterinarian.

CHAPTER 2

In January, with only four and a half months of clinics left before graduation, my classmates and I began to explore what our first jobs as veterinarians might be. I sat at the rickety kitchen table in the wreck of a house I shared with five other women vet students in West Philadelphia, trying to ignore the cockroaches rustling in the paper bags stored between the fridge and the sink. The "veterinarian wanted" advertisements in the back of the *Journal of the American Veterinary Medical Association*, known as JAVMA, were arranged by state and practice type. I circled all the listings for large animal vets in upstate New York. Paging through to the section on internships, I stumbled on a listing. It was a clinical internship at Utah State University, where my friend Nancy worked.

Nancy had been assigned to be my "big sister" my freshman year of veterinary school, when she was a sophomore. When I first saw her with her fringed leather jacket and blue jeans, hands stuffed in her back pockets, big grin on her face, I had a feeling we would be friends. Nancy was not ashamed of skipping out on studying for a beer or a joint. She made sure I knew where the best parties were on weekends. She graduated in 1977 and started a job in a pathology lab. Even in Utah, where alcohol was scarce and weed scarcer, she managed to find a group of friends. She dated a cowboy, which seemed like a natural thing for Nancy to do.

I gave her a call.

"Nancy, it's Linda."

"Linda! What's going on?" She sounded just the same, and I smiled, remembering our crazy partying.

"Listen—I'm job hunting, and I saw the USU internship listed. It's large animal, right? You think I should apply?"

"Sure, why not?" she said. "But what about Vincent? Aren't you going back to Freeville after graduation?" Nancy had been a sympathetic ear when I was lonely in Philadelphia. She knew my years away from Vincent had not been easy.

"You know I want to do large animal medicine, and I've got a bad feeling about those dairy vets in upstate New York hiring a woman."

"You think you would move to Utah?"

"Probably, if it was my only option, and just for a year."

"So go for it, although I have to tell you, these Mormons were okay with me doing the laboratory work, but a clinical internship?" She sighed. "They just don't get women doing what they're sure is a man's job."

I wasn't surprised when I didn't hear back from Utah State.

I passed the National Board Exam, required for a veterinary license, but I still had to take a licensing exam in the states in which I wanted to practice. In late March, I mailed my application for the New York State exam given in mid-May, just after graduation. By then I hoped to have my first job near Freeville lined up.

Veterinary practices that need another vet know when to list their jobs in JAVMA—senior vet students looked for jobs in March and April. By May, most positions for new graduates were filled. I set a juice glass full of cheap red wine on my bedside table, propped the pillows against the wall, and again flipped open JAVMA to check the large animal job listings. There were a dozen listings for large animal jobs in rural New York State. I circled each one, imagining those farm boys at Cornell Veterinary School and how they would be looking at these jobs too.

I closed the journal and grabbed my juice glass. I needed another drink, and I didn't want to miss *Saturday Night Live*, the new comedy show. Too late now to call any of these practices anyway. I just wouldn't think about the possibility that for me to get the job

I had trained for, Vincent and I would have to part again. I didn't have to make that choice yet.

❖

Large animal veterinarians were difficult to reach by phone that spring before graduation, plus I had little time between clinical rotations to make calls. They worked from five a.m. to early evening, driving their white vet trucks from farm to farm. Most had a receptionist who took their calls, booked appointments, ordered the drug inventory, and handled the business side of the practice so the vet could concentrate on the patients. Not uncommonly, this person was the Wife. The Wife wasn't eager to give her husband a message that a girl had called about the job listing. The Wife was hoping for a big, strong man to help out with her husband's backbreaking work—someone who could take over a chunk of the practice so that maybe her husband could get home before the kids were in bed. The Wife couldn't envision a young woman in this role, and besides, why on earth would a woman want to work in such a rough and dirty job? My messages were often "lost" or ignored, and I called again, sometimes three or four times, before a message would make it to the busy vet husband, who might call me back for a short telephone interview.

It took four calls to finally get Dr. Patterson in Skaneateles, New York, on the phone.

"Dr. Patterson, I'm calling about your ad in JAVMA."

After a beat of hesitation, Dr. Patterson said, "Yes?"

"I'm graduating in a few months from Penn, and the ad says you would consider a new grad for the position," I said, my voice high and nervous.

"Penn, you said?" Dr. Patterson was most likely a Cornell grad who didn't have a lot of respect for the Penn training in dairy medicine. "What's your name, young lady?" From his gritty voice, I pictured Dr. Patterson as a middle-aged, heavy-set large animal veterinarian. I gripped the phone and pushed on.

"My name is Linda Rhodes, and yes, Penn," I said, in a rush, "but I spent a summer in Ithaca, milking at the Cornell Dairy, and then the second summer I rode ambulatory with the Cornell vets." Ambulatory is the part of veterinary training where students ride with professors in vet trucks, going out to farm calls. The summer after my sophomore year, I participated in an exchange program at Cornell Vet School. Penn students came to Cornell for cow experience, while Cornell vet students went to Penn to learn equine orthopedic surgery.

Likely the Cornell Dairy did not count as real experience to Dr. Patterson. Most local dairy farmers thought the Cornell Dairy was run by a bunch of elitist PhD types who didn't know the front end of a cow from the backside. Rumor was that the dairy sucked up a big budget but the cows had unimpressive milk production.

A long pause from Dr. Patterson. I sat silent, waiting.

"Well, young lady," he chuckled, "I have a couple of men from Cornell coming up for an interview." I scowled at the phone.

"But I'm happy to take your phone number." I wound the long, black phone cord around my arm and paced.

"Dr. Patterson, please. I'll be in the area next weekend, and it would be great to meet you." Skaneatlas was an hour north of Freeville, a hard commute but possible.

Dr. Patterson cleared his throat. "Well, dear, it's nice that you want to work up here, but the winters are pretty rough. Maybe I can get you up here sometime in the summer, and we'll see how things go."

My counterfeit laugh filled some space.

"I grew up in Rochester. I'm used to snow," I said, my voice ridiculously high.

"Okay, then, I'll let you go," he said. And he meant it.

❖

Some veterinarians promised to call back after hearing from a few more people. Some said thank you, hung up, and never returned follow-up calls. Many told me flat out that they wouldn't hire a woman. But once in a while I was invited for an interview. Much later I came to realize that the interview invitations were extended only by the most desperate veterinarians—the ones who hadn't had a vacation in seven years; the ones with clients who milked fifteen cows in a broken-down parlor and paid their bills late or never; the ones with practices in the far north where the snow could reach six feet in the winter and their truck started only if a little heater coil was inserted in the oil pan; the ones who couldn't attract a Cornell man to their practices. No one else would apply for those jobs. They might have to make do with the girl vet.

So I went. I borrowed my sister's car to drive to remote practices in places like Penn Yann, Oneonta, and Watertown. Tiny upstate New York towns, surrounded by miles of green, rolling hills, oak woods, fields dotted every half mile with tall blue silos full of corn silage, gray barns with rusty weather cocks turning in the wind. Miles and miles of winding, unmarked roads dotted with dairy farms. Everyone knew everyone, and not just by name—by the model of pickup truck, by the day they came to the local grocery store, by the teachers their kids shared in school. Cows fueled with corn silage and timothy hay cut fresh from the meadows made the milk that was the river on which these communities floated.

In March and April, the raw spring months before graduation, I went north on weekends to find a job, squeezing in travel between clinical assignments and studying. I was a woman in a man's world. Many times, in many ways, I had been told I did not belong. But I showed up anyway, not expecting much of a welcome. I launched myself on my chosen path, blasting into an unwelcoming universe, fueled with hope and determination.

Most of these men had never seen a woman large animal veterinarian. I had the good luck to study with Dr. Elaine Hammel at Penn, an accomplished large animal vet who did farm calls. I rode with her every chance I could get. The vets who were recent Cornell graduates had worked with, or at least known, Dr. Mary Smith during their ambulatory rotation. She was a young woman vet whose father had taught at Cornell and was one of two women graduating from Cornell in 1972. Now she was a resident, working in the department that did farm calls, and during my summer at Cornell, Dr. Smith took me with her. She was confident and accomplished in the dairy barns. The dairymen considered her kind of a freak of nature. Plus, she was an academic veterinarian, not a "real" practicing vet, and even worse, she was interested in goat medicine. Goats were a backyard hobby animal, not like dairy cows, the economic engine of the local farms.

I didn't give up hope. I knew I was smart, graduating *summa cum laude*, fourth in my class. I had spent my summers with cows. I had grown strong with the hard, physical work we did in clinics and could hold my own in the barn. The argument that a girl was too weak to do the job made no sense to me. I weighed about a hundred and thirty pounds; a big Cornell farm boy might weigh two hundred pounds, and a large dairy cow weighed over fifteen hundred pounds. Wits and good sedative drugs were more important than muscles.

I could tolerate a low salary, tough working conditions, and punishing hours. Just a few weeks working with them would demonstrate how much I could do, how hard I worked, how good I would be for their practice.

CHAPTER 3

IN EARLY APRIL, I VISITED a practice near Canandaigua, New York, for an interview with Dr. Sherman. His practice was farther from Ithaca than I wanted, but it was getting late into my senior year. I needed a job. He was a country vet, dirty truck, the Wife. He had graduated from Cornell fifteen or twenty years earlier, a time when women, with few exceptions, were not admitted.

With my work clothes, stethoscope, bandage scissors, thermometer, and rubber boots in the car, I drove through the early-morning countryside of upstate New York, rolling hills, pastures just beginning to green, spring sunshine warming the dark soil, the air so fresh I could eat it. A welcome relief after the grime of Philly. The sun was in my eyes when I turned northeast, toward Canandaigua, window down, tapping out a beat to Jackson Browne singing "Running on Empty."

Down a long driveway ending at an old farmhouse and classic red hay barn, I saw a vet truck, full of drawers and equipment. Dr. Sherman came out his front door and shook my hand firmly.

"You made it," he said, walking toward his truck. "Let's get going."

He pulled into the driveway of a run-down farm with dead tractors, broken harrows, piles of rubble scattered in the yard. No one was around. On a sunny spring morning, the farmer and farm-hands were out on their tractors preparing the fields for planting.

"Got this call yesterday. A bull needs a ring in his nose," Doc Sherman said. The bull, the farmer had told the Wife, would be tied up in the shed.

Dairy bulls are amazing creatures. Lovely at birth, they weigh a mere hundred pounds and have large liquid brown eyes, extravagant eyelashes and soft black noses. But they grow rapidly into huge, ferocious beasts, powerful beyond belief with murderous intent for anyone who would merely walk by, much less attempt to perform a medical procedure.

The nose ring is one way to control these raging maniacs—a typical rope halter would not suffice. Pulling on a rope tied to the nose ring is painful for the bull, allowing a handler some measure of control. Walking toward the shed, I remembered watching Dr. Hammel do the procedure on a young bull my senior year. The ring opens on a hinge to reveal a sharp pointed end on one side. Dr. Hammel leaned up against the young bull while I held the halter, stretching the bull's neck out. In one decisive move, she pushed the ring through the nasal cartilage. It reminded me of a human ear piercing. Quick and painful. The bull let out a bellow, and it was over.

In a young bull weighing up to six or seven hundred pounds, no problem. But when Doc Sherman and I walked into the shed, I could see that our patient was much bigger. Maybe a thousand pounds, shoulder as high as mine, head as big around as a large exercise ball, rump about three feet across. He was all black with a little white patch around one leg like a sock, and he was furious. Fully sexually mature, with hormones showing, he was used to being out in the pasture, mounting his girls. But today, all morning, he'd been rudely confined to this little shed, waiting for the veterinarian to arrive. He panted, bellowed, pawed the ground, showing his masculinity. He rolled his eyes and tossed his massive head around, spittle flying. He was only a teenager (on his way to a fully mature two thousand pounds), but he knew something was up, and he was not going to like it.

The small shed was in terrible shape, knocked up with rough two by fours, a tarpaper roof, two small stalls inside, separated by quarter-inch plywood. It must have been built for sheep at one time, or perhaps for the kid's 4-H ponies. It looked like the next big wind would topple it. This amount of bull was too much for such a rickety structure, and the bull seemed to know it.

Doc Sherman handed me the ring and a halter, said, "Go ahead," and stood off to one side.

I put the halter over my shoulder, took the ring, and looked at it. Time seemed to slow down, and I cautiously walked toward the bull, trying to think. Shouldn't we tranquilize this creature? Dr. Hammel didn't use a tranquilizer when she did the procedure, but that bull was half the size of this one. I looked back at Doc Sherman, and he smiled and made a little shooing motion with his hands. The bull spotted me and perked up his ears in my direction.

My heart started to pound. I looked again at the ring in my hand and stopped for a minute. I was on a job interview. Was I supposed to be able to do this? Could a big man veterinarian do it? Could Doc Sherman do it?

Don't climb into the pen, I thought.

I tossed some sweet alfalfa into the feed bunk, and when the bull stuck his head in to sniff it, I threw the halter over his head, cinched it close, and ran the free end around the post on the side of the stall. He bellowed in surprise. I tied a slipknot, restraining his big head, and reached in my pocket for the ring. This might work out better than I expected. With the bull's eyes bulging and protruding tongue dripping saliva, I grabbed his head and, with all my might, pushed the sharp end of the ring against his nasal septum. He jerked his head in pain. His skin was so tough that the ring didn't penetrate, but slid off the slimy surface, leaving a raw red scrape. Now he was seriously mad. He jerked his head back and the two-by-four post that he was tied to snapped in several places like a dry twig. I was holding a slimy ring, and the bull was tied to a loose piece of lumber about a yard long, with splintered ends, which he swung in all directions as he tossed his head in fury.

With a guttural roar, he crashed through the feed bunk and came after me. I ran flat out, made it to the fence, leaped up and had one leg over when he crashed into my other leg, smashing it between the fence and his enormous forehead. I managed to pull free and land on my side in the dirt on the right side of the fence. The bull lost interest and trotted away. Liberated, he headed out to the pasture to his ladies, wearing the halter and a piece of the shed, ringless. I lay on the ground breathing heavily, leg throbbing, heart racing, and glad to be alive.

Doc Sherman chuckled. I lay there for a minute, waited for my heartbeat to slow down, my leg already swelling. Gingerly, I tried to put weight on it and winced. It hurt, but I could walk—it wasn't broken. My side where I landed was covered with dirt. I shook clumps of mud out of my hair. Balancing on my good leg, I leaned on the fence and brushed off the worst of the grime.

"Now how do you plan to get that piece of wood and rope off him?" Doc Sherman said, still grinning.

I stared at him, feeling the throb in my leg with each heartbeat. A crow cawed and flew over the shed. There was a long pause. He mumbled something about another call and that he would come back later for the bull. He walked back to his truck. I hobbled along, climbed in, and tried to stretch out my hurt leg, but the cab was too cramped. I looked forward to some ice and aspirin. The ride back was silent. Tears pooled in the corners of my eyes, but damn it, Doc Sherman would not see me cry.

When we arrived, he hopped out of the truck, slammed the door forcefully and disappeared into the office without a word. I got out, dragging my swollen leg, and awkwardly wiggled out of my coveralls and boots.

Goddamn it, at least he's got to say something before I leave. I hopped over to the office, went in, and eased down into a chair by the door. I had so hoped this might be the job I was desperate for, and I had blown it.

There was no sign of Doc Sherman.

I looked around. A heavy black phone and an answering machine sat on an old wooden desk scattered with slips of paper—bills, maybe, or notes of calls. Dirty linoleum floor, a two-year-old calendar with a picture of a cow on the wall. God, my leg hurt. My eyes started to burn, and my throat tightened up, when a door in the back opened and a sturdy-looking, middle-aged woman poked her head in.

"You want some lunch?" she said. "My husband had to go out again, but I have some sandwiches made." I gulped and wiped my eyes with my dirty sleeve.

"Sure, can I take a sandwich with me?" I asked. She nodded and came back with a brown bag. I guess this meant the job interview was over.

"Ham and cheese," she said. Her nails were bitten, and she wore a floral-patterned housedress and slippers. "Hope that's okay?"

She watched me struggle to my feet and handed me the bag. "And a cookie," she said, smiling.

"Thanks, kind of you," I said.

"Okay, then," she said, backing up toward the door.

❖

When I arrived home, Vincent was sitting on the back porch, playing his mandolin and humming a tune. I limped over and sat on the steps.

He put the mandolin down. "How'd it go? You okay?"

"Horrible," I said. "Got my leg smashed up."

I wriggled out of my jeans to see the extent of the damage. Above my knee, a dark purple-blue bruise extended to my hip, swollen and angry looking. I was glad the bull had missed my knee joint.

"That looks nasty," Vincent said. "What happened?"

"Get me some ice to put on this, and I'll tell you the whole story," I said. I limped into the house in my underpants and flopped down on the couch.

He came back with a dishtowel wrapped around some ice cubes. I scrunched over so he could sit next to me.

"Honestly, Vincent, I'm worried that none of these guys will hire me," I said.

He shrugged and patted my good leg.

"No, really," I said. "Most of them don't even want to meet me, much less hire me." The ice melted and dripped on the couch. I wanted to get in the shower and take a handful of aspirin. My leg throbbed.

"Something will turn up," he said. He picked up his mandolin. On my way to the shower, I heard him singing "Oh Death" in the living room.

What is this that I can see, with icy hands taking hold of me?
I am death and none can tell, I open the door to heaven and
    hell.
Oh Death, O Death, please spare me over till another year.

CHAPTER 4

AFTER THE BULL INCIDENT, I was careful not to try anything dangerous again. I visited at least ten practices in New York that spring,
from Honeoye, west of Canandaigua, all the way east to Cazenovia
south of Syracuse, with the same depressing outcome.

"You know, honey, you really have some pretty good qualifications," another vet said. "If it was up to me, I'd hire you, seeing as
I'm so busy and could use some help, but my wife, you see, well,
she doesn't really feel comfortable with the idea of me working
with a woman in the practice."

Another month went by, and again I was searching the next issue
of JAVMA, sitting at my ratty kitchen table in Philly. A three-man
dairy practice, good salary, just down the road from Freeville, in a
little town called Dryden. Perfect—we wouldn't have to move, and
I would make enough money to be able to pay my student loans
and have a life with Vincent.

The next morning, I called the number early, hoping to catch
the vet instead of the Wife. "Let this be the one," I prayed, dialing
the phone. Luckily, the vet picked up.

"I know they're graduating women from vet schools these days,"
he said, "but I've never seen a girl do large animal work."

I sat on the floor of my bedroom in Philadelphia, holding the
big black receiver to my ear.

"But I . . ." I started to explain my experience.

"I just can't see how you could do it," he interrupted. "I'm a big
guy, and sometimes I have a hard time pushing those cows around."

"I can come up to your practice and spend a day on calls," I said. "I could come next week."

"Thanks, dear," he said. "I don't think so."

By May 1978, with senior year almost over, most of my classmates had found positions. The men interested in dairy cattle had jobs in good practices scattered throughout rural Pennsylvania. The upstate New York dairy jobs, as expected, went to Cornell men. By May, with graduation looming, I had $28,000 in student loan debt, with payments due four short months away.

My plan seemed simple enough. I wanted a profession that combined science, life in the country, and a reasonably secure income. Vincent and I were apart for four long years. We had expected that after I graduated, we could make a life together somewhere in upstate New York, each of us living our dream. I knew that few women practiced dairy cattle medicine, but I also knew it could be done. Look at Dr. Mary Smith at Cornell and Dr. Elaine Hammel at Penn, two women who had taught me so much. Someone had to give me a chance. I was running out of options.

I began to rethink my career strategy. Maybe I had to look farther afield, knowing that meant asking Vincent to move away from everything he loved. California surely was a more liberal, looser place—the land of the hippies, the beaches, the flower children. Maybe California dairy veterinarians were different, more willing to consider a woman large animal veterinarian. And my parents lived in Altadena. I could stay with them while I looked for a job.

If Vincent wouldn't come to Philadelphia, I knew it was crazy to think he might move to California. When I applied to take the California Board Exam, I didn't tell Vincent. That conversation was too hard just now. After so many years of keeping this relationship alive, and four years living apart, was it time to let it go?

❖

Before I fell in love with Vincent Abruzzo, I fell in love with my guitar. The old, beat-up nylon-string guitar that I found at a garage sale was good company for a lonely young teenager in 1964. Using a chord book and lots of patience, I taught myself a few folk songs, pretending I was Joan Baez. When I was a junior at Eastridge High School in Rochester, New York, I grew my hair long and straight and begged my father to take me to the 1965 Newport Folk Festival. One hot July afternoon, I sat on the grass listening to Joan Baez and mouthing the words I had memorized from her album. Scandalously, Bob Dylan horrified the folk purists by singing "Like a Rolling Stone" backed up by electric guitars.

In the lonely summer of 1967 after my freshman year at Sarah Lawrence, I worked at a bleak office job and went home to dinners with my parents. I picked out old folk tunes on my guitar, singing them to myself late at night. At folk festival gatherings, I connected with other college-age kids who played folk music—and would later be called hippies. Somehow I found myself in a little band with a couple of long-haired guys, standing on a washtub bass in an orange miniskirt, singing Jim Kweskin jug band songs. We crooned "Ukulele Lady" and "Somebody Stole My Gal." I couldn't get enough of it. I skipped work to rehearse and signed up for every gig I could. That's where I met a band that played lightning-fast bluegrass tunes and Doc Watson–style folk music. All three brothers in the group played anything with strings—mandolin, guitar, fiddle, banjo—and sang harmony. Vincent Abruzzo was my age, the oldest of the three.

Vincent's band was a bunch of talented, goofy musicians. They fascinated me. I had a crush on all of them, but mostly I was attracted to Vincent. His wild, curly black hair stuck out in a halo around his head. He had deep brown eyes decorated with ridiculously long eyelashes. About my height, he was slim, with strong hands that flashed over his guitar strings—gentle, delicate, and precise—making music. I loved his clothes. Worn blue jeans, loose cotton shirts with no collar, dark silk vests. He wore jaunty caps and John Lennon glasses.

His fingertips were calloused and hard from hours of making music on steel-stringed guitars. With graceful and gentle hands, he touched me like he touched his instruments, making music. One late night that summer, I lost my fingers in the thickness of his black curls when we kissed in my parents' living room, wishing we could take off our clothes. Josie, my mother, coughed quietly, signaling she could hear us.

Vincent pulled back. "I should probably go," he said. "Your parents are awake."

❖

For privacy, we necked in Vincent's parents' Rambler parked in our driveway, steaming up the windows while we listened to Van Morrison sing "Brown Eyed Girl." We were all in love, in love with the scene, the music, the rush away from the conventional world of our parents into an alternative culture. When I think back on that time, I don't remember why I picked Vincent, in particular. Maybe it was because he paid attention to me, attention I needed like a wilted plant needs water. He almost never spoke, his silence suggesting some profundity I didn't understand, deep as a black-watered forest pond. Whatever it was, we fell in love. At bonfires on humid summer nights, we sat in the flickering light and sang. I watched Vincent lean back against a log, fingers flying over his guitar strings, and wondered how I was so lucky to have him love me. He and his band, the brothers, the coolest scene in Rochester, and I was a part of it.

Never mind that I would never be a cheerleader or a join a sorority like my sister, Anne. Never mind that I didn't get invited to Princeton football weekends like my classmates. Now in my small world I felt loved and safe and pretty. Vincent touched me with his gentle gaze, and my loneliness evaporated like mist. He held me in his calm arms and gave me sweet kisses. I went back to Sarah Lawrence a little less lonely.

I didn't think about marriage or forever, and deep down I thought I needed more than Vincent could offer. Maybe that's why I set off for California after graduation, the summer of 1970, flinging open the door to wider possibilities. Rochester and Vincent were safe, while California was risk and excitement. I was ready. I don't remember saying goodbye, but I must have, and it must have been sad. We made no promises, except to write a postcard now and then.

CHAPTER 5

I DIDN'T GROW UP ON a dairy farm and I never rode horses, although I loved watching Dale Evans ride her buckskin horse as she and Roy Rogers sang "Home on the Range." In fact, my only exposure to animals when I was a child was our pet cats. I was certainly not one of those kids who always knew she wanted to be a veterinarian. In college, I wasn't interested in studying biology and concentrated on math and physics. I didn't have any idea that I had vet school in my future when I graduated from Sarah Lawrence. I was off on an adventure, with no particular goal in mind except exploring a wider world.

In the spring of 1970, Nixon bombed Cambodia, and anti–Vietnam War sentiment exploded. My male friends were terrified of getting drafted since student deferment had been scrapped. Campuses erupted in protests, classes were canceled, and antiwar protesters blocked traffic on bridges into Manhattan—students were even gunned down at Kent State. We were protesting the war in Vietnam, helping young men burn their draft cards and escape to Mexico, writing manifestos, and protest marching. Nothing was normal.

What we started calling the "counterculture" was blossoming. We stayed up late thinking great thoughts about alternatives to the nuclear family and what we might do instead of working a deadening corporate job.

After graduation in May of 1970, Vincent had a year of art school to finish, but I was about to graduate and ready to explore a wider world. The idea of staying in Rochester to be near him didn't cross my mind. We searched for alternatives to the stultifying

suburban world of our parents. My sister, Anne, had married her
college sweetheart, Bob, a son of a banker. After serving a couple
of years in the Peace Corps, they ended up in California, living an
alternative lifestyle on a commune, a movement that was taking
hold in rural areas all across the country.

"Do you have a job lined up?" Anne asked.

"Haven't even started looking," I said.

"Come to the west coast," she said. I could hear the excitement
in her voice. "It's amazing."

❖

The farmstead was purchased by two of Anne's wealthy lesbian
classmates from Vassar—two hundred and fifty acres of magical
redwood forest with a run-down house, a teepee, and a large
barn. They called it a commune, I guess, because most things were
shared. There were sheep, milk goats, a couple hundred chickens,
a donkey, a horse, a dog, way too many cats, and a big vegetable
garden. Carmen and Jeanne were learning to live off the land.
Jeanne was in charge of the animals, and Carmen baked bread in
the old wood cookstove, spun and weaved the sheep's wool, and
made cheese from goat's milk.

A college friend from California offered me a ride across the
country, and we headed west. I was excited to be on my way to
the epicenter of the counterculture—northern California. I wasn't
interested in the conventional expectation—get a job, rent an apartment, marry, have kids. Instead, I would get back to the land, grind
flour for bread, grow vegetables, gather eggs from the chickens,
and experiment with free love and vegetarianism.

❖

The farm was as amazing as Anne had said. Everything was new
to me, and I got up every day excited to learn new skills—how
to shear a sheep, milk a goat, split wood, drive fence posts, and
stretch field fence. We made butter and cheese from goat's milk,
baked bread in a woodstove, and read the Whole Earth Catalog,

looking for encouragement in our back-to-the-land efforts. I was terrified of the chainsaw but impressed that Jeanne was not. I'd never seen a woman wield a chainsaw.

We started a woman's consciousness-raising group, smoked dope, and went naked to get comfortable with our bodies. I took the only mirror in the house down, put it in the attic, threw out all my makeup, and stopped wearing a bra.

The boundaries of our previous suburban, nuclear family culture of the fifties and sixties cracked open, and the cornucopia of alternative possibilities of the seventies poured out. Communes spread among the redwood forests and windy shoreline of Route 1 in Mendocino County. We were the flower children, fluid groups joining, dissolving, reforming, free of the need of permanence, going with the flow, being here now. We explored new ways of living, sang new songs, and took new lovers, left them, and loved others. We danced naked in the misty redwood forests, swam in psychedelic rivers.

My connection with Vincent grew thinner, more tenuous, as we had no phone, and our only communication was through the occasional letter. He moved to a commune in Nova Scotia. Our relationship was in hibernation.

❖

The goats started it. They fascinated me. I learned about breeds—Nubians with their long floppy ears, white Saanens with their short legs, brown-and-white Toggenbergs with striped faces, each with her own personality. Smart, mischievous, prone to escape, the small herd of twenty goats was not enough to be a commercial dairy, but it was a great source of milk, yogurt, butter, and cheese for us, with some left to give away. Our small library of goat husbandry books and the *Merck Veterinary Manual* taught me about parasites and worming, abscesses, and mastitis. The goats themselves taught me that slowing down and observing was the key to knowing when something was normal and when to call the vet. After almost a year of caring for the goats, I still had so much to learn.

One day in August, I went to the barn for the early-morning milking. It was already hot, and the air was still, straw chaff floating in the shafts of sunlight; a rooster's crowing echoed. Irma, the big Nubian goat, eagerly jumped onto the milking platform to gobble sweet oats and molasses. I sat down on the milking stool and washed her udder with a damp rag. She shifted her feet and munched loudly.

"Okay, Irma, girl, just relax," I crooned. Her udder felt a bit warmer than usual; the milk that squirted from her left teat was watery, with yellow flakes. I saw a few specks of blood. Irma stomped her foot and shifted away.

"I know, I know it hurts," I said softly. "We've gotta get all that nasty stuff out of there." Gently, I milked out the teat—the cup of liquid looked more like serum and pus than milk. Jeanne walked in the barn, a shovel over her shoulder.

"I think Irma has a problem," I said, holding out the cup. Jeanne took a look and wrinkled her nose.

"Ugh," she said. She fetched the thermometer and sure enough, Irma's temperature was 104.5 degrees, a couple of degrees higher than normal. "I guess I could give her some of those antibiotics we had left over from the last time."

"Call the vet," I said. "Let's do this the right way." My shoulders tensed. I shoved my hands in my overall pockets. Jeanne didn't like being told what to do.

The vet arrived in the late afternoon, a trim, middle-aged guy with large hands and ropy muscles. He headed to the barn, and I followed. Jeanne wasn't around.

The goats cocked their ears forward, watching the vet.

"You the owner?" he said, turning to me.

"No," I said. "I help take care of them. I live here."

"What's the problem?"

I explained what I'd seen. He looked back at the goat herd.

"That big, brown Nubian?" he said. "The one over by the fence?"

"That's her," I said. How did he know?

"Okay, let's get her up on the milking stand."

A scoop of grain in Irma's feeder enticed her to cooperate. The vet did a quick physical, head to toe, stethoscope, thermometer, running his hands over her back, checking each of her feet. I watched as he squeezed a milk sample into a metal cup with a strainer. The milk was yellow flecked with small red clots of blood. It smelled rotten.

He stood up, put his hands on his lower back, stretched and sighed.

"Good you called. Mastitis can get pretty bad quickly."

I followed him out to the truck and watched as he took out a small brown bottle, some syringes and needles, half a dozen antibiotic tubes to stick up into the teat.

"We'll start her on injectable antibiotics as well as some in her teat," he said as he drew up some yellow fluid into a small syringe and attached a needle.

"You can give the follow-up shots, right?" he said. I felt my stomach turn over. I had never stuck a needle in anything.

"I'll show you," he said, noting the panic on my face.

He explained that the shot would go deep in the muscle of her back leg and showed me how to restrain her by climbing up on the milk stand and leaning my full weight against her rump. My heartbeat quickened, and I had that metallic taste in my mouth that precedes vomiting.

"Here you go," he said, handing me the syringe. "Don't worry. She won't feel it much—it's a small needle."

"Don't think about it, just jab it in hard right here," he said, pointing at the upper back part of Irma's left leg.

Gulping deep breaths, I leaned over, thrust the needle and felt it sink into the muscle surprisingly easily. Irma jumped a little but didn't struggle.

"Good. Now slowly push the plunger."

The yellow liquid flowed out of the syringe until the plunger was all the way down. I jerked the needle out, making Irma jump again.

"Do that once a day for five more days, and alternate back legs," he said, tearing the wrapping off a mastitis tube. "This part is easier. Milk her out completely, put the blunt end of this tube into the teat and slowly push the plunger." He demonstrated, and Irma didn't even flinch.

"Do that after every milking until all the tubes are gone."

After the shot in Irma's leg, the udder stuff looked easy.

"Don't drink the milk for five days after the last treatment. You don't want an antibiotic milkshake," he said, grinning. The sun was low as we walked back to the truck.

"Keep those syringes in a clean place," he said. He brushed his boots with disinfectant. "Keep an eye on the other goats—it can be contagious. And be sure to wash your hands between goats when you milk." The big truck's engine roared to life.

"If her temperature isn't down by tomorrow afternoon, call me again," he said as he leaned out the window and looked directly at me. I was smiling and nodded solemnly.

After a dinner of lentil soup and brown bread, I found an old copy of the *Merck Veterinary Manual* and read the section on mastitis a couple of times, not understanding half the words. The fat book was ripe with information. I read sections on intestinal parasites and exotic diseases like foot-and-mouth, so named because it caused nasty blisters on both the feet and mouths of animals. Science—I missed science and technical knowledge. We tried to take good care of our animals, but in reality we knew almost nothing. There was an abundance of knowledge to be had, and I wanted to have it.

I climbed into bed that night and stared at the ceiling, hands behind my head. I had a growing realization that I was tired of communal living. Most of the time and energy was soaked up with growing and preparing food and chopping wood for heat. The hard, physical work left me too exhausted to even read a book in the evenings, and certainly no time to think about the science I loved. And worse, us communal folk, who were supposed to share everything and work together, bickered about who had left the barn door open, who slept late and avoided the morning water hauling, and whose turn it was to clean the outhouse, the most hated chore. I was sick of having no money. But I loved the farm and the animals. I still felt giddy from giving my first injection! Look at that vet—he wasn't sitting behind a desk, he was on farms all day, physically active, helping animals and making a living. Plus, he could do all kinds of wonderful things that would be exciting to master. The logic worked—it felt right. I would be a large animal veterinarian. Now I just had to figure out the path. I yawned. How hard could it be?

❖

Anne and her husband moved to Santa Fe, where Bob got a job in an art museum and Anne got pregnant. In 1971, she had a baby girl named Satya. She tried to make a life with Bob, but the role of housewife and mother wasn't a good fit.

"She's finally down for a nap," Anne said. I had called to wish her happy birthday. "I'm exhausted. How's things in California?"

"Kinda tired of communal living," I said. I pet Bamboo, the Siamese cat curled up on the chair next to me. "Trying to figure out what's next."

"Me too," Anne said. "Bob gives me no help with Satya. He's at work all day, and I'm stuck in the role of wife and mother." She sighed.

"I feel pretty stuck here too," I said. "Probably time for me to think about what's next."

I heard Satya cry and call for her mother. "She's up. Gotta go."

❖

After the morning milking, I sat on a hay bale in the sun, back against the worn barn boards, sipping coffee and imagining going back to school. Sitting behind a desk wasn't what I wanted in a career. I loved the past year of physical work, outdoors, getting strong, learning new skills. Honestly, I wanted both independence and some regular income. I was sick of being dirt poor. Putting this all together, becoming a large animal veterinarian seemed like the perfect career. Science, outdoors, physical labor, a profession that I could practice anywhere there were large animals, and a steady income. I had no idea how to make a large animal veterinary career a reality instead of a passing fantasy. I let it go, for the moment. There was no one to tell me that getting admitted to veterinary school was difficult. I would soon find that out.

My parents, Dusty and Josie, always supported my wild ideas, and it would be good to explore this particular crazy idea with them and hear their reaction. Next time I was in town, I called them from a pay phone. The rest of the commune didn't need to know my plans yet.

"I think it's a great idea," Dusty said. It felt so good to hear his reassuring voice.

"I don't know if I could manage sitting in a classroom again," I said. I pushed another quarter into the coin slot. "Plus, I would have to take some biology courses just to apply."

"It's been two years you've been there. Sounds to me like you are tired of the commune world," Dusty said. "A challenge is just what you need. Here, talk to Josie."

I told her what I was thinking and how sick I was of being poor and directionless.

"And what about Vincent?" she asked. "He's still in Rochester, right?" Vincent had given up on his commune in Nova Scotia and was back in Rochester playing music with his brothers.

"I miss him. I miss the music too." I put another quarter in the slot.

"So just come home." I could hear her smile. "You can stay with us until you figure out what you want to do."

Outside the phone booth, the sun was going down. I needed to get back to the farm for the evening milking.

"I'll think about it."

By the time I got back to the farm, I knew the answer.

CHAPTER 6

I RETURNED TO ROCHESTER AND to Vincent, who had grown a big bushy beard and an impressive mustache. I was unsure of what might come next but grateful for his sweet smile and gentle touch. We connected as if a few years were a few weeks, and I was back in his heart and he in mine.

I moved into my parents' Rochester home. My sister and I called our parents Josie and Dusty instead of Mom and Dad. We were used to it, but our friends still found it odd. I once asked my parents if they had formulated any child-rearing rules. Josie explained that they had agreed on two rules when my older sister, Anne, was born in 1945. First, they wanted their children to call them by their first names—Josie and Dusty—instead of Mom and Dad because they wanted us to think of them as people, not just parents. Second, they intended to walk around the house with no clothes on and not lock any doors, so that their children would be comfortable with naked bodies.

Vincent's family was first-generation Italian. Ida and Vincent Abruzzo Sr. had five children: Vincent Jr.'s two younger brothers, Frank and Anthony, also musicians; an older married sister; and a bedridden, profoundly disabled sister, whom Ida lovingly cared for at home. Ida went to Mass several times a week. Vincent's father ran a small local grocery store with his brother, a butcher. Their extended family was large, loud and loving, and expected each son to settle down, marry, have a gaggle of children, and buy a house down the street so the grandparents, aunts, and uncles could hold them close, and they could all work in the grocery store Vincent's father ran.

Vincent and I didn't talk much, but we understood our relationship wasn't going to be like that of our parents. We didn't want monogamy—we wanted freedom. Maybe that's what made it so exciting—we took nothing for granted, each kiss important. We agreed our relationship would be open.

On a hot summer day in 1972, I sat on the lawn at an outdoor festival, listening to the Abruzzo brothers play. When his set was done, Vincent found me waiting backstage. He traced the edges of my lips with his finger. I looked into his deep brown eyes and sighed.

"I missed you," I said. He leaned in for a kiss, his mustache tickling my lips.

"Glad you decided to come back," he said, brushing the hair off my forehead.

I quit my waitress job and spent the summer painting houses with Vincent and his brother Frank. We fell back into our familiar attraction, and Vincent and I were a couple again.

"What do you think about getting an apartment?" I asked. Vincent and I were perched on ladders next to each other painting porch trim a deep blue.

"You think we could afford it?" Vincent asked. He dipped his brush in the gallon can. "I don't have much saved up."

"We could find somewhere cheap. I don't care if it's funky." I pushed the hair out of my eyes and felt the sweat dripping down my back. "I'm so tired of sneaking around to sleep together."

"Sure," he shrugged. "We can at least look."

The local paper listed some inexpensive apartments in downtown Rochester that might be suitable. I didn't realize that an Abruzzo family crisis was set in motion when Vincent's parents found out.

"I heard you two are looking at apartments," Vincent Sr. said. He put down his fork and pushed away his plate, red with a little remaining pasta sauce. I was at the Abruzzo family Sunday dinner, sitting next to Vincent, who looked down at the tablecloth.

"Is it true?" His father was staring at us, and Vincent shrugged.

"Don't shrug at me!" Vincent Sr. shouted. He pounded the table, making the dishes clatter. I jumped. I'd never seen him angry.

"In this family, if you live together, you live together as husband and wife." Ida grabbed some dirty dishes and retreated to the kitchen. Vincent sat stock still, wordless.

The Abruzzos could not abide sex without marriage. After all, what would the aunts and uncles say? How could they explain it to their friends? What a disgrace to the family. But I could not abide marriage. My world was still the hippie commune free love world, even though for now we were a couple. Our compromise was a wedding on paper only. I didn't change my name, we didn't exchange rings, there was no ceremony, no dress, no gifts, no flowers. Only a brief signing of legal papers. I think it broke Ida's heart, but at least she didn't need to be ashamed in front of her relatives.

❖

I pretended nothing had changed. Of course, even if I refused to call him "my husband" and wouldn't allow him to say "my wife," the undertow of thousands of years of culture swept me out to sea. I navigated, but the current dragged me places I had not expected to go. Not that I became a housewife, but I found myself being jealous when groupies crowded around Vincent after a concert. *He's mine*, I thought. We became a couple, when before we had been free to roam on our own. We never did rent that apartment. Even if we pooled our meager earnings, we couldn't afford it.

I still had my dream of a career as a large animal veterinarian. The brochures from Cornell and the University of Pennsylvania described in detail the prerequisites for applying to their veterinary schools, the cost and the procedure for submitting an application. At a minimum, I would have to take organic chemistry and three biology courses. Even the application fee seemed out of reach. For now, I put the dream aside.

Vincent's band decided to rent a house, live together, and try to earn a living making music. He wanted to play music with his brothers and a few other musicians who had played off and on together for years in Rochester. Maybe if we pooled resources from a larger group, we could afford rent somewhere. When I talked to Anne about it, she admitted she was ready to leave her dysfunctional marriage and might be interested in moving east to join us.

In 1973, the year the Watergate scandal broke in Washington, a motley group of eight people came together. My sister, Anne, and her daughter, Satya. Vincent's middle brother, Frank, with his wife, Kathleen. And Anthony, Vincent's youngest brother, had fallen in love and brought his girlfriend along too. With few plans and less money, we all decided to live together, sharing our resources in a setting where the band could play gigs. We found a dilapidated old house in Hop Bottom, Pennsylvania, where we could live for free in exchange for taking care of the property. Free was perfect.

In college I had studied "intentional" communities of like-minded people that formed to forge an ideal alternative living arrangement. B. F. Skinner's *Walden Two* was popular then, describing a utopian community of free love and non-nuclear families. Ours was more an unintentional community, with no rules, no plans, no structure. The band took over the living room. Drums, guitars, mandolins, fiddles, and banjos were scattered around, along with empty beer cans and cigarette butts. We pooled our money for groceries and gas and shared the use of a lime green VW bus that Frank and Kathleen had bought with their wedding present cash. Waitressing at a local diner and working at Elk Mountain Ski resort as a ski rental girl for minimum wage plus tips bored me to tears, but it gave me plenty of time to think—and I thought again about applying to vet school.

CHAPTER 7

I LAY ON THE BED in the cabin, windows open to the breeze off the meadow, and stared at the ceiling. I thought about my interview at Penn vet school, how thrilled I was to get accepted, and how hard it was to leave for Philadelphia, knowing Vincent was staying in Freeville with his band. Four tough years apart, the grinding work of veterinary school. How excited I was to graduate, how much hope I had. Now my dream of taking care of cows in upstate New York had died.

"You packing?" Vincent asked, his big brown eyes downcast, his long lashes shadowing his cheeks.

"Taking a break," I said, sitting up and stretching. I planned to stay with Josie and Dusty while I looked for a California dairy cow job. They'd moved to Altadena from Rochester after Josie was diagnosed with aggressive breast cancer during my first year of veterinary school. After her awful chemo and radiation, they decided another winter in Rochester was too hard, so Dusty transferred his Xerox research to a lab in Pasadena, California. His work developing the first color copier was going well, and Xerox was happy to accommodate him.

"Not much to pack," I said.

Green coveralls, stethoscope, bulky knee-high rubber boots, along with a couple of heavy textbooks, a few t-shirts, and pairs of jeans, overstuffed the suitcase. I zipped it up, heaving it to the floor with a grunt. Vincent sat on the edge of the bed, staring at the floor.

"California boards are the middle of June. Everyone says they're easier than New York boards," I said. The cabin was hot, the air sticky, the scent of wet grass on the breeze. Flies buzzed around the open window. I glanced at Vincent. His shoulders drooped. He sat still as stone.

"I'll keep looking for jobs here," I said, and sat down on the bed next to him. "You never know, something might turn up."

He flopped down on his back, put his hands behind his head, and bent his knees into a V.

"What are you thinking?" I asked.

He shrugged. This was the least productive question of our marriage, but I kept asking it. Neither of us knew, exactly, what we were thinking. Now, in the middle of June, student loans about to come due, just when we hoped we could settle down to our new life, I would be three thousand miles away from Freeville.

❖

My parents' house in California was a retro, art deco–type structure in Altadena, a sprawling pin oak in the shady front yard. With big windows, an overgrown garden with lemon trees, the house was perfect for them. I lay in the guest room, sprawled on the bed, after my long flight into Los Angeles International and the traffic-clogged drive.

"You okay?" Dusty asked. He had lugged my heavy suitcase through the garden and up to the guest bedroom.

"Tired. Long day," I said.

"Get some rest. Josie's making dinner," he said, brushing my hair off my forehead, like he used to do when I was a child. The guest room was a calm space, with wheat-colored walls and a bright quilt in a modern design Josie had folded on the bed. A brown ceramic pot she'd made held a bouquet of black-eyed Susans. After a nap and dinner, we opened a bottle of Dusty's homemade red wine and caught up on the news of old friends. None of us wanted to talk about the job search or about Josie's breast cancer, in remission since her diagnosis and treatment four years earlier.

I was blessed with parents who were perfectly happy with me choosing whatever path I wanted. They valued independence and nonconformity. Dusty was a photographer, a researcher, and a professor, but most of all, a thinker. Josie was a housewife. She used her creative energy to make fabric art and ceramic pots. I was proud of her social justice work in the Black community in Rochester.

Both my parents had been raised dirt poor in tiny Colorado towns, Dusty in Crawford, a rough cattle-ranching town on the western slope of the Rockies, and Josie in Platteville, a town known for sugar beet farms, on the flat fertile plane to the east of the mountains. After my sister, Anne, and I were born, they came east so Dusty could study photography at the Rochester Institute of Technology, paid for by the GI Bill. They dreamt of a wider world, travel, art, music, and books, and eagerly left their rural Colorado roots behind to try to scramble out of poverty. Josie subscribed to the *New Yorker* and splurged on classical music concerts at the Eastman School of Music. Dusty was employed at the Graphic Arts Research Institute experimenting with inks and printing technology, so excited with his work he spent weekends in the darkroom and laboratory, often with me and Anne in tow. His friends from the lab hung out in our shabby living room to smoke cigarettes, drink wine, and talk philosophy and politics late into the night. Dusty set up our slide projector and a rickety roll-up screen to view photographs they'd taken that week. Josie served homemade banana cream pie and percolator coffee. I fell asleep stretched out under our round dining room table, listening to their animated conversation and laughter.

I'm sure Josie and Dusty were pleased that I had found a career path and was accepted at an Ivy League veterinary college. But honestly, I knew they would have been just as pleased if I became a plumber or an artist or anything, if what I did made me happy.

Over the next week, I lazed around their garden, lemon and avocado trees shading the intense sun, the scent of citrus in the air. I thumbed through the June issue of JAVMA, checking listings for both New York and California. All the California jobs were for small or exotic animal practices. No listings for dairy vets. I had already contacted all the New York listings—there was nothing new.

June was blistering hot in southern California; thick smog blanketed the valley. The beach was a long traffic jam away. I was out of money, with no car, no job, and an expensive veterinary degree that I could use only in New York State.

The California Board Exam started early and was over by noon. A few weeks later, when I opened the test result envelope and saw my passing grade of just over 70 percent, I felt my whole body relax; I'd been in a semi-clenched state since that awful exam. I heard that half of the UC-Davis grads had failed.

Now that I could practice in both New York and California, I had nothing to do but look for a job.

❖

Josie brought in the mail. "This what you've been waiting for?" she asked, handing me the new issue of JAVMA. I flipped to the back pages where the jobs were listed by state. There was a California dairy vet job listed—just one. "*Veterinarian wanted for position in busy four-man dairy practice. Proficiency in reproductive work a must. Weekend and emergency work required. Experience preferred but new graduates considered.*"

I thought about the repro lab junior year at Penn, remembering being up to my armpit in a cow's rectum, trying to feel the uterus and ovaries. Proficiency was a stretch, but at least they would consider a new grad. The practice was a four-hour drive north of Altadena, in the flat central valley, land of the big dairy farms. A receptionist answered my call. I was relieved to deal with a professional—no Wife in evidence. After taking some basic information—I'm a new graduate, yes, I have a California license, yes—she said she would check and call me back. Within the hour, she did, and I was invited to interview.

Josie overheard the phone call. "Your California job!" she said, grinning.

I shrugged. "I'm not getting my hopes up."

I was used to small, picturesque red barns, cows neatly stanchioned side by side, happily chewing on silage with the milking machine whooshing in the background. Cows were often called by name: Suzie, Spotty, Molly, Jessie. California dairies were milk factories, identification numbers tattooed on the cow's sides.

Josie smiled. "But a cow is a cow, right?"

❖

The receptionist said I would be working with Dr. Richmond for the day. If he was favorably impressed with me, I would come back to meet the other vets in the practice. Driving out of the lush subtropical June heat of Altadena, over the dry scrub-covered mountains, I repeated the job description in my head: "Proficiency in reproductive work a must." I knew what it meant. It meant rectal exams. I remembered Dr. Bartholomew's coaching on how to feel the uterus and ovaries of a cow through the rectum. He was one of the experts in dairy reproduction at Penn.

"This cow is about sixty days pregnant," Dr. B had told us. He stood behind her, holding her tail curved over her back, with his arm up to the shoulder in her rectum, and his chest pressed against her backside. "Once you get proficient at a sixty-day pregnancy diagnosis, you'll want to work at getting that down to forty days or so."

I pulled a long plastic sleeve on my left arm and squirted it with some lube. Dr. B pointed to the cow next to him. "Try her. Tell me what you feel."

As soon as my arm slid into her rectum, she began straining. I raked the manure out of her rear as my arm started to go numb. The slimy rectal tissue slid around when I groped for the uterus. I wanted to feel something, anything definite, but it was a big mush in there. Dr. B said, "Think of the anatomy, Linda. Feel for the hard cervix, then run your hand forward to the uterus."

The cow and I both strained and grunted. The armpit of my coveralls was covered in manure, the sweat ran down my back. Dr. B shook his head. "Take a break," he said, probably because he felt sorry for the cow rather than me. My classmates and I named these palpation sessions "hope and grope" because no one reliably identified any anatomical structure.

Dr. B explained, while we washed up, why this was so important for dairy cow reproductive management. "Remember, it's a cycle. Cows need to deliver a calf before they can make milk. Gestation is nine months." He leaned against the sink and stripped off his coveralls.

"If the farmer can get his cows pregnant within sixty days of calving, that cow will be optimally profitable for him." The farmer was always a him. "It's our job to see if his cow is pregnant. If she is, he is all set. If she isn't, then he needs our help to figure out what the problem is—and quickly."

I learned that a cow comes into heat every twenty-eight days. Heat is when, to put it bluntly, she wants sex, and she makes that pretty clear. She sniffs other cows' rear ends and restlessly paces around the pen looking for a bull. She will mount other cows, pretending to be the bull looking to breed, and then she will reverse the role and stand stock-still while another cow jumps on her rear end and pretends to breed her—this is called "standing heat."

"It's not only pregnancy diagnosis," Dr. B said. "When you get proficient, it's important that you help the dairymen figure out the best time to breed a cow." He sat on a hay bale, pulled off his rubber boots, and stretched. "A lot of the bull semen these guys use to artificially inseminate their best cows is expensive."

I had read about the investment market in bull semen—but only for sperm from elite bulls. These elite bulls, with names like Kingboy, Mogul, Dragonheart, and Defiant, had daughters that produce large amounts of milk.

"You ever have to treat dairy bulls?" I asked.

"Rarely, thank God," Dr. B said. Those animals are hard to handle. "Even for a routine foot trim, you have to knock them out."

❖

Driving into the Central Valley, I saw fields of sweet peppers, corn, and tomatoes unroll in neat rows. My shoulders were so tight they almost touched my ears. I shook out one hand and then the other to relieve my fingers, cramped from clutching the steering wheel.

I thought about the men who now were successful practitioners but once had exactly the same dilemma I did. None of them were born with their arm in a cow—they had to learn too.

In Dr. Richmond's office, I sat on a metal chair holding a paper cup of hot black coffee, on time at seven a.m. Dr. Richmond, after politely inquiring about my trip and commenting on the weather, cleared his throat.

"How many rectal exams are you comfortable doing in a day?"

"Well, as a new graduate, I haven't had the opportunity to do more than about twenty at any one time." I shifted in my chair, trying not to be discouraged. He furrowed his brow.

"I'm eager to get more experience, and I'm sure that with some intensive practice in this position, I'll catch on quickly," I said.

"Dr. Rhodes, my men and I do over two hundred rectal exams each day." He took a sip of his coffee from a white mug with a tractor supply logo on it and looked out the window.

"We work in rough conditions. You know summer here in the Central Valley is hot as the dickens, way over a hundred degrees in the barns."

He leaned on his desk. "Have you been here in the winter? Well, of course you haven't. It rains for weeks at a time. The barns fill with shit up to the top of your boots."

We looked at each other. I crossed my legs and smiled, trying to look friendly.

That seemed to irritate him. "This is rough stuff, little lady."

Dr. Richmond was about five feet, two inches in his manure-stained socks. His blond hair was cropped short, face clean-shaven and pale, his arms muscular. He lifted his chin and drew his eyebrows together. He was just getting warmed up. He paced around the office, wagging his finger like he was scolding a kindergartener.

"I already knew how to do a thirty-day pregnancy check when I graduated Davis."

He was right in front of me now, looking down.

My face flushed and my armpits dripped under my coveralls. Dr. Richmond walked to the door, opened it, and stood there.

"Thanks very much for coming, but this is not the job for you. It's too bad my receptionist didn't have me speak directly to you on the phone. I could have saved you the trip."

I stood up, stunned. "Okay, well, thanks."

My car was broiling hot. I rolled down the windows, took a deep breath, and pulled out of the driveway. I drove the slower back roads to Altadena, not in a rush, until the sunset and the stars came out over the desert. On the way, I stopped for some sour cherry pie at a roadside diner, went into the restroom, and had a good cry. I was out of options. I flipped on the radio and found a country music station with some cowboy whining about how his honey walked out on him and he felt like crying and dying.

New York, California, and Wisconsin were the three big dairy states, and I'd tried to find a job in two of them. Attempting Wisconsin would mean I would have to move again and take another state board exam. I couldn't face another failure in another state. Plus, I was broke. In two months, my student loans were coming due. The moon rose, the stars gleamed in the deep black sky over the farm fields, and the road spooled out in front of me.

❖

My parents saw the look on my face when I arrived late that night, and they didn't even ask. They weren't used to seeing me discouraged. Josie poured me a glass of Dusty's red wine. I sat at the kitchen table and felt my chest constrict. Tears streamed down my face. I swallowed a sob. Giving up suddenly seemed like a possibility. Josie handed me a tissue and stood behind my chair, hugging me with one arm and leaning her cheek on my hair.

The next morning, I dialed Freeville from the kitchen phone and sat on the tile floor.

Anne picked up.

"Vincent's fast asleep. Had a late-night gig and got home at three a.m. How's California?"

"It's okay, Josie seems to be feeling good."

"That's a relief. And what about the job scene?"

"Horrible. Absolutely no luck."

"Only one interview, and the little twerp of a vet told me women can't do the job."

"Did you punch him?" she laughed.

"Felt like it."

"Vincent will be relieved. He wants you to come home."

"Come home to what?" I asked. "No jobs there. You know how hard I tried." I stood up and stretched my back. "Just tell him I called," I said.

"Sure, will do, give Josie and Dusty hugs from me."

I went to the backyard, lemon scent strong on the gentle breeze, my bare feet warm on the stone steps. I thought about Vincent, playing his guitar, his gentle fingers moving gracefully over the strings, making music together with his brothers. He had found his home. I wished I had. My old dream of being a large animal veterinarian had started in California, back in 1970, on a goat farm. Could this be the end?

CHAPTER 8

JOSIE FROWNED AT HERSELF IN the hall mirror as she applied her bright red lipstick. She ran a comb through her short graying hair. "I hate these appointments," she said.

She was going to her oncologist at the Huntington Hospital in Pasadena. Today was her next visit to check for any evidence of her breast cancer. She had been scanned every six months for over four years now, and each time the news had been good, but it didn't get easier.

"Want me to drive you?" I asked. The hospital was on the far side of Pasadena, a long, traffic-intensive drive, and I had nothing to do.

"No, you stay here," she said, snapping her purse shut. "If it's bad news, I'll need time to process it." Always a mother, protecting her daughter.

"It'll be fine." Hugging her close, I could feel her uneven chest. She had decided not to have a breast reconstruction after the mastectomy. "You've been clean for four years."

She pulled back, brushed the hair off my forehead and smiled. "I know, I can't help but worry."

❖

I remembered when I first got the news about her breast cancer in October 1974, just after I had moved to Philadelphia to start vet school. Josie's general practice male doctor had been telling her for months that her symptoms were just menopause—the pain under her arm, the tiredness, finally her breast pain. By the time she went to a woman doctor for a second opinion, her cancer was so advanced the doctor diagnosed it as soon as Josie took off her blouse. She was in surgery that week. The cancer had eaten into her sternum and spread to her lymph nodes.

The earliest I could get home to Rochester after the surgery was Thanksgiving of my freshman year. Josie had lost weight, her movements stiff and awkward. Her surgical wound had not yet healed, and she fretted about cooking the traditional Thanksgiving dinner. Even rolling the piecrust took too much energy. She didn't protest when Anne and I took over.

I could help with wound care, or at least everyone thought I could now that I was learning medical stuff. Each night before bed, Josie and I retreated to the bathroom, where she sat on the toilet with the lid closed and took off her shirt. Shocking how much weight she had lost. Her chest was oddly out of balance with one droopy breast, and on the other side, a raw wound six inches long, extending from her sternum to her armpit.

"It hurts," she said. "I take a pain pill an hour before the bandage change."

"Have you been doing it yourself?" I asked.

She nodded. "Dusty hasn't seen it. I don't want him to see it until it's healed." Her forehead was crunched into wrinkles, blue circles under her eyes. She instructed me in the bandage routine. Josie looked away; her shoulders pulled up. She had been an energetic, beautiful woman, voluptuous, with clear white skin and big brown eyes, bobbed dark brown hair in waves. Now her body prematurely aged, her skin fragile and dry.

"Does it hurt?"

"Not too bad," she lied.

I dried her chest with cotton balls, squeezed a bit of triple antibiotic ointment onto my index finger and gently applied it to her incision. I covered the wound with sterile gauze, wrapped a cotton bandage under her arm, over her shoulder, and around the wound area in layers, not too tight. I felt her relaxing. She shrugged awkwardly back into her blouse.

"Good as new!" she said brightly, but standing up, she swayed on her feet, woozy from the pain and the pain meds.

For Thanksgiving, we each gave thanks that Josie had survived the surgery. Dusty drank too much red wine. Anne and I went for a walk in the cold, silent woods behind our house and cried. Josie napped in the afternoon and went to bed by eight, exhausted. Sunday morning, she was up early, sitting in the big, black leather chair in the kitchen with a mug of hot coffee, looking out the window at two exquisite white-tailed deer, browsing in the yard. She smiled, put a finger to her lips, and pointed out the window. I sat down on the broad arm of the chair, she put her hand on my knee, and we watched the deer together.

❖

Once her wound healed, Josie endured several rounds of radiation and chemotherapy. Then we had good news that the scans indicated the tumor was gone, and other than monitoring for metastasis every six months, Josie could resume her normal activities. But there was nothing normal about surviving such an invasive cancer and its brutal treatment. Josie's energy was fragile, and the things she had once enjoyed—entertaining friends, cooking, sewing, making pots on the potter's wheel in the basement—now seemed impossible. She drank coffee, read books, watched the deer out the kitchen window, and rested.

So Josie wouldn't have to endure the isolation and stress of winters in Rochester, Dusty was pleased to work with Xerox to move his research lab to their location in Pasadena, California.

Anne and I didn't hear about their plans until everything was settled. Our parents were moving to Altadena and selling the quiet house in the woods where we grew up. They planned to move in the late spring of 1975. Josie's oncologist had recommended a good doctor there, and Dusty was already shipping equipment to his new lab.

Studying helped me ignore my worries and focus on the vast amount of material I had to memorize. In December of 1974, the end of my first difficult semester, I called Vincent, hoping for some comfort.

"Linda!" He sounded glad to hear me.

"Vincent, hey."

"You okay?" Vincent asked. I seldom phoned because of the cost of a long-distance call.

"I need you to come down." All I heard on his side of the line was a sigh. The silence went on a beat too long. "Please, I need you here. Josie is sick, and vet school is crushing me." I waited. More silence. I thought about how nice it would be to get back from classes and be greeted by a hug and a hot meal.

"Vincent? Are you there?"

"Yeah."

"What do you think?"

"I just can't, I told you already."

"But I need you. I'm so lonely. Just come down for next semester, and then we can be in Freeville for the summer." I waited, hoping he would understand how difficult it was to ask like this, to plead, really.

"Linda, it just doesn't work for me." I held the heavy black receiver to my ear. There was another beat of silence. "The band is finally getting gigs," he said.

I felt my chest tighten and my eyes burn.

"We've been writing a lot of new music."

Now it was my turn to be silent. I was angry that he wasn't willing to help me, and immediately guilty that I was asking him to leave what he loved.

"And what would I do all day in the city?" he said.

Tears dripped down my face, and I needed to blow my nose. My hands trembled holding the phone. I gave up. "Okay."

CHAPTER 9

DUSTY WAS A THINKER, A down-to-earth, practical, problem-solving guy, helpful in any situation. He could lift the hood of a stalled car and spot the loose wire, or crawl under the sink and find the leak. He saw the problem—his daughter badly needed a job as a veterinarian, and it had been almost four months since she graduated. Although he didn't know any dairy vets, he did know the vet who cared for his beloved cat, Polo. Within a few days, Polo made an unnecessary visit to the Pasadena Central Veterinary Clinic.

The sun streamed in the living room's big picture window. I curled up in the black leather chair reading a vet journal, a fuzzy white goat-hair rug under my bare feet. The pin oak tree by the driveway drooped, baked in the sun, dry and dust covered.

"How was the checkup?" I asked.

Dusty's eyes softened, and a corner of his mouth turned up in a smile.

"Polo's fine." He put his arms around me and pulled me close to his heart. "She's overweight, from too much pampering." I lay my cheek on his chest, listening to his slow, steady heartbeat. Polo meowed loudly from the kitchen. When Dusty opened a can of tuna for her, I pushed my hands in the pockets of my shorts, waiting.

"Busy practice," Dusty said. "Waiting room was packed." He fussed with the tuna can lid, draining the juice.

"I told Dr. Jacobs about your job hunt," he said, spooning tuna onto a plate. Polo circled between his legs, purring loudly. I plopped down on a kitchen chair and kicked my flipflops off to feel the cold tile under my feet.

"So he knows I have no job prospects," I said. Polo gobbled the tuna from her little cat dish. Dusty walked over to me, put his warm hand on my shoulder and sat in the chair next to me, his knees almost touching mine. He leaned in, his face close. I could see the gray hair in his eyebrows.

"He's looking," Dusty said.

"Looking for what?"

"Another vet. He said he'd like to talk to you."

I shrugged and pushed my chair back a few inches. The energy drained out of my body. Dusty reached out and patted my knee. Polo finished her tuna and jumped on the table, washing her whiskers with her paw. Dusty waited. I scratched a mosquito bite on my ankle and looked at him. We both knew the deal—I was out of money, loans coming due, and zero dairy vet job prospects.

"Maybe," I shrugged. I went through the sliding glass door to the garden and sat down on the bench by the shed. Sun glowed through the dappled shade, warming my back. The dry leaves of the avocado tree crackled softly in the breeze. I stared at the lemon tree for a while. Lemons on trees still seemed weird to me.

We both knew I wasn't coming back to Freeville, but I dreaded telling Vincent about a possible small animal job in Pasadena. I couldn't tell him. At least, not yet.

❖

I made an appointment to meet Dr. Jacobs and see his practice. He was a trim guy, in his late forties, with a jaunty style—bow tie, light pink shirt. His office was piled with veterinary journals on the desk, walls covered with thank-you notes and cards with pictures of dogs and cats he had treated. Textbooks overstuffing the bookshelf, a dog bed in the corner, a chewed green leash hanging from the doorknob.

He offered me a job and I accepted. My loans were due, what choice did I have?

"As long as you understand I'm going to keep looking for a large animal job. I can't make any promises about how long I might stay."

"Fine with me, just as long as you stay through the busy summer." He reached out his hand to shake mine, and just like that, I had my first job.

On the way back to my parents' house, driving through the freeway traffic, I rolled the windows down to feel the hot Southern California wind, tuned into a rock and roll radio station, and sang along. *You can't always get what you want, but sometimes you get what you need.*

❖

I treated a big Labrador for diarrhea after he'd raided the garbage. The yowling young female cat that the owners thought must be in terrible pain was actually in heat. They were so relieved you would have thought I'd cured their cat's cancer. The owners of a lame bulldog expected a diagnosis of arthritis or worse; instead, a grass awn had burrowed into the tissue between his toes and caused a draining abscess. Tweezers and a foot soak solved the problem. This small animal practice gave me more satisfaction than I had expected, and I surprised myself by being pretty good at it.

I'd been working a few weeks when my first challenging case showed up. A young California couple, both tan and blond, wearing shorts and tie-dyed t-shirts, carried a chocolate Labrador puppy wrapped in a pale blue blanket.

"We found him this morning, lying on his side in his puppy bed," the young man said. The woman's eyes were red—she'd been crying. I laid the droopy little puppy, tiny ears and tail hanging down, on the table. When I touched his belly, he shrieked a high-pitched squeal. The woman winced. I felt a hard lump in the puppy's abdomen. It was likely a piece of bowel telescoped in on itself, not uncommon in puppies, called an intussusception.

"Your puppy has a serious intestinal problem and needs surgery," I said, in a calm voice, trying not to alarm them.

"Oh no!" the woman said, scooping up the puppy and holding him against her chest.

"It looks like you caught it early," I said. "If we get him into surgery today, he should recover just fine, but of course, it all depends on how bad things look when we open him up."

"Okay, doctor, whatever he needs." The woman nodded vigorously.

"We love this little guy," the man said.

The puppy's gums were pale. He was dehydrated. I took him in the back, where the technician started him on intravenous fluids. As I scrubbed my hands with disinfecting soap, I tried to remember—sometimes, it was possible to gently pull the telescoping bowel apart and it would heal on its own. But sometimes, if it had gone too long, a section of bowel would have to be removed and the ends stitched back together, a surgery I had watched but never done.

Lucky for this little pup, once he was under anesthesia and I opened up his belly, I was able to gently pull the hard, bright red piece of bowel back into shape. The angry red faded quickly, and the piece of bowel turned a healthy pink.

After stitching the layers of the abdominal wall and the delicate puppy skin, I pulled the tracheal tube out of his tiny mouth and took him into the recovery area, where he lay still on his blanket next to a hot water bottle. By the time I changed out of my scrubs, he was holding up his small brown head.

For the next few days, I hung out with my patient. I took him out of his cage and sat on the floor with him resting in my lap, while I checked the stitches on his belly, happy to see everything held together, healing as it should. After surgery, in every case, the intestines go quiet for a while; nothing moves. I listened with my stethoscope for sounds of the bowel gurgling and growling—sounds that incidentally have a wonderful onomatopoetic name: borborygmi. Most importantly, I waited for the patient to poop.

The next day, I checked the puppy every half hour, hoping for the first post-surgical poop. The poop watch. The little guy looked good, but what was going on inside? Was the bowel breaking down, leaking toxic fluids into the abdomen, soon to kill him, with his current good recovery short lived? He needed to poop! One day went by, then two. Waiting for dog shit—what had my life come to? He ate, drank, bounced around in his cage, licked my hand. Where was all that food going? It had to come out the other end, didn't it? If it spilled out his damaged bowel into his abdomen, he'd look sick, wouldn't he? With my limited experience, panic was just under the surface. On the second day after surgery, in my parents' living room reading a novel before bed, I obsessed about the puppy. I had to know—had he pooped yet?

The house was quiet. Josie and Dusty had gone to bed. I grabbed my purse, slipped on my sandals and went out. The air smelled of lemon trees and desert wind. Up here by the mountains, the air was cleaner than in the valley. I took a deep breath. After the short drive to the practice, I turned on the lights in the quiet clinic, a couple of cats in cages, recuperating from being spayed, fast asleep. When I got to my patient's cage, I saw the sleepy little guy. He looked up at me trustingly and whacked his tail on the bottom of the stainless steel cage, proud of himself. And yes, there it was: a large, glorious, bowel-shaped, fully formed poop. The puppy jumped into my arms when I opened the cage and licked my face. Who would have thought dog poop would be such a cause for celebration?

❖

I was a doctor, practicing medicine, making good money, paying off my loans, like a grownup. I had almost decided to adopt an orphaned cat named Spot who lived in the practice. But I lived with my parents, my husband was three thousand miles away, and I couldn't shake the feeling that I was in a holding pattern, waiting for my real career to start. Josie cooked, Dusty and I talked about things we enjoyed: Freud and dreams, intuition and mathematics, logic and riddles. We drank wine and ate fresh avocados. Josie and Dusty played tennis. I read novels and studied my veterinary textbooks when I had a puzzling case. We enjoyed one another's company and avoided the hard conversations. What about Vincent? How long would Josie's remission last? Would I ever get back to the cow barn?

July in Pasadena started a run of brutally hot months. I thought about calling Vincent or writing him a letter, but really, what was there to say? Long-distance phone calls were expensive. I flopped down in the black leather chair and stared out the window. I had no friends to meet, no errands to run.

"Why don't you see what's on PBS?" Josie said, looking up. "Maybe there's a nature program."

"Not in the mood," I said, flipping through some records. I put Dave Brubeck on the turntable.

"I'll do the dishes," I offered. "Maybe I'll bake a banana bread."

"You okay?" Josie asked. How did she always know when something was going on with me?

"I was just thinking. I miss Vincent."

She nodded. "It must be hard," she said. She took off her glasses and wiped them with her shirt.

"You think he'll come out to California?" she asked, turning to look at me.

"We haven't figured that out yet. He doesn't want to." I couldn't imagine that Vincent and I would settle down in Altadena, with me working in a small animal practice and him three thousand miles from his brothers and his band. In the spring, I would turn thirty, and I felt like nothing was certain, my relationship on hold, no friends, the job I hoped for eluding me. How could it be that I had become a practicing vet but felt almost like a failure?

"Something will happen." Josie reached over and patted my shoulder. "You know me, I have good intuition." It was true, she did, but I couldn't imagine what that something might be.

By the time the banana bread was cooling on the kitchen counter, Josie and Dusty had gone to bed. I lay flat on the couch, watching a moth flutter around the ceiling. Polo saw it too, and we kept each other company, watching the moth bump up against the light fixture, trying to get out where there was no window.

CHAPTER 10

ONE MONDAY, I FOLDED LAUNDRY and listened to Joni Mitchell sing about putting up a parking lot. I heard the phone ring.

Josie called, "Linda, it's for you!" Only Vincent called me at my parents' house, but he usually called on Sunday when the rates were cheapest.

"Linda, hi!" A familiar woman's voice, but I hesitated to place it . . . wait . . .

"Nancy! Wow, how did you find me?" It was my "big sister" from Penn, the hard-partying cowgirl.

"Yeah, hi!" she said. "I called Vincent, and he gave me your parents' number." Hearing her voice brought back some great memories of fun parties and watching *Saturday Night Live* with my roommates in vet school.

"So, are you done with Utah?" I remembered her working in Utah. Something to do with pathology maybe?

"Just wrapping up," she said. "What a place. I'm looking forward to getting out of Dodge."

"What's next?" I asked.

"Moving back East. I'm gonna study public health. Got into a master's program."

"What happened to the cowboy?" I didn't remember his name, her boyfriend in Utah.

"We're kind of on hold. He's headed to Alaska for a big oil job," she sighed. There was a story there, but before I could ask, she said, "Linda, I've got an idea for you." Since we were talking boyfriends, the thought crossed my mind that she meant a cowboy just perfect for me, too. "The Utah State clinical internship job is wide open. They're looking for a new grad for that position."

"A new grad? Didn't they fill that position last spring?" Thinking back on the application I sent in back in March for that job, I realized that I'd never received a response.

"They did. Hired a big, blond guy, new grad from Colorado or Washington State or somewhere."

"Figures," I said. "Bet he was a Mormon."

Nancy laughed. "Yup, for sure." Okay, this wasn't making sense. They filled the job, but it was available? "I remember you applied for that job last spring."

"I never heard back from them. I'm sure being a girl didn't help my chances," I said.

"Anyway, of course they hired a Mormon guy."

"Of course," I said.

"He left the end of June, and the position is open."

"Left?" I said. "What happened?"

Nancy chuckled, "I shouldn't laugh, but I heard he got kicked by a cow—both his legs broken."

"Wow, broke both legs!"

"They had to drag him out of the barn, I heard," she said. "I think they took him down to the hospital in Salt Lake."

"Too bad. I bet it was quite the spectacle."

"That's why I tracked you down. You really ought to apply for that job." Nancy knew how much I wanted a cow job.

"I'm not a blond Mormon guy who grew up on a dairy farm."

"But you have a good chance," she said. I leaned into the phone and felt a small bit of hope blossoming in my chest.

"How's that?" I asked.

"The position is only for a new grad, and all the vets from the class of '78 already have jobs."

"So what? They'll find some good old boy," I said, not wanting to want this job.

"I know, I know," she said, "but they are pretty desperate at this point."

"Why's that?"

"They need someone to do the work, and what's his name, the golden boy, has been gone since June."

"Did he really break both legs?"

"Crazy, right? Pins and screws and casts and everything," she said. I started to think she might have a good idea.

"Let me think about it," I said.

❖

A Utah State internship was not the job of my dreams. First, it was in a university setting, and I longed for private practice, working directly with the farmers. Second, it was in Utah. Vincent would hate the idea. Third, with my sex, drugs, rock-and-roll hippie background and feminist attitude, it seemed crazy to think about living in Utah's Mormon world. I called Nancy back.

"Who should I contact about that internship?"

"You should call Dr. Nelson. I've got his number right here. He's a nice guy, old-fashioned Mormon, salt of the earth."

"Oh geez," I said.

"Yeah, I know. But give it a shot."

"Okay, I just might do that. Nancy, you are a true friend. I'll keep you posted."

I hung up, and Josie looked at me and winked. I was already dialing the Utah number. I listened to the phone ring, my breathing shallow and fast, my palms damp.

"Dr. Nelson here." There was a pause, and I launched into my pitch.

"Dr. Nelson, Dr. Nancy Hilber gave me your name."

"Oh, Nancy, sure," he said. "I know her from the pathology lab."

"Yes, and she told me how much she enjoyed working with you," I lied. "She said you might need someone for the clinical internship?"

"Yup," he said, and there was a pause.

"I applied for that position back in March. Maybe you remember? My name is Linda Rhodes, I graduated from Penn vet school last May. I understand it's a job for a new graduate. I'm very interested in this position and I was hoping you could tell me what I need to do to apply for it." I heard myself talking too fast.

"Where did you say you went to veterinary school?"

"University of Pennsylvania. Graduated summa cum laude."

I held my breath to stop my speed talking and waited for him to say something.

"Nancy tell you about the unfortunate accident?" he asked. "Shame that young man won't be in shape to work for quite a spell." There was a long pause.

Finally, he said, "You understand this job requires working with cattle?"

"Yes, that's exactly why I'm interested. My veterinary training has been focused on dairy cattle."

"We've decided to re-advertise the position. We need to evaluate some new applicants. You should see the ad coming out next week."

"I already know I want to apply," I said. "Can you send me an application now, or maybe you can get the one I sent last March out of your files?"

"Oh, we discarded those after we selected Dr. Johansson for the position. What a shame that young man couldn't finish out the year." Another heavy sigh followed by a loud creaking noise. I could picture him leaning back in his office chair.

"Losing that young fellow was tough. You know, we have a big dairy farm, and over four hundred head of beef cattle, plus a large collection of quality sheep and goats. Taking care of this bunch is running me ragged."

"That's a big responsibility," I said, thinking, if only I could keep him talking, maybe I could progress this a bit farther. "It must be hard to cover the emergencies."

"Yeah, that's the hardest part. My wife's not used to me going out on a calving anymore. Those middle-of-the night calls are the worst when I have to work the next day." I clucked my concern. He continued, "You know, it's really gonna be tough when I have to start teaching in September."

He spoke with a soft drawl, not Southern precisely, but a quiet and pleasant accent that I came to know was characteristic of a Utah native. I let him talk.

"Last week I had to preg check over a hundred heifers, it was hot as the dickens, and then, just after I got cleaned up and settled down to eat supper, the dairy's best cow came down with milk fever, and I had to run back down to the barn."

This sounded like my dream job.

"My wife was not pleased. It was Prayer Night at the Temple."

I had no idea what Prayer Night at the Temple was. The chair creaked again. I was standing with the phone pasted to my ear, trying to think of what else I could say that would get Dr. Nelson to invite me to Utah. The silence became uncomfortably long. I finally spoke.

"Dr. Nelson, I'm qualified for the position, and I'd like to come out to Utah to talk to you about it. I'll send you my résumé, and then maybe we could make plans for me to come and interview next week."

"Well," he said, and there was another long pause.

"I could start right away, and I'd be happy to cover your emergencies."

He chuckled. "My wife would be grateful. I'll have to think it over, talk to the department . . ." he trailed off. I could hear the rejection building up in his head. "A girl! My friends at the university will laugh at me for even considering it. I would have to hold her hand all the way! Couldn't possibly work."

I pressed on. "Dr. Nelson," I pleaded, "no obligation. I'd be happy to come out just to meet you and see the university and your fine animal science program. I've heard a lot about it." I never knew Utah State University existed before Nancy told me about it.

"Let me have a think on it. Appreciate you calling," he said. "Tell me your name again?" I spelled it out, and gave him my phone number, too. We said goodbye, and Josie came over and put her arms around me.

"See?" she said. "I told you something would turn up."

CHAPTER 11

A COUPLE OF DAYS WENT by. Late into each night, my stomach knotted, I lay wide awake. I slaved over my meager résumé and sent it to Dr. Nelson overnight mail. What else could I do? I had practically begged for an interview. It was eight hundred miles from Altadena to Logan, Utah, and I wanted to jump in the car and just show up.

After a week, I couldn't stand it anymore. I called again.

"Dr. Nelson, this is Dr. Linda Rhodes. I sent my résumé last week. Did you get it?"

"Yup."

"Did you have a chance to speak to your colleagues about my interest in the position?"

"Yup, sure did." I watched Polo walk into the kitchen to check for leftover crumbs in her food dish. Again, the sound of the desk chair creaking. I offered, "I could drive to Utah next week, to meet with you."

Dr. Nelson cleared his throat. "Well, Linda, I guess it couldn't hurt to talk to you, if you want to make the trip."

I took that as a yes, and we set a date for the next week. My hopes, trampled under far too many rejections, were close to dead. But here was a tiny seed of possibility—a seed that could sprout and grow into optimism. I would be crushed by another rejection—possibly the end for this career path. What the hell. At least I would see some lovely country on the drive.

I told Dr. Jacobs I was headed to Utah for a job interview. Knowing where my heart was, he was happy to see me excited. I called Nancy—she let out a whoop.

"Yahoo! Come on out to Utah! You're gonna love it."

"Whatever happens with this job, at least we'll get to visit."

"I'll try and get a few of my non-Mormon friends together for you to meet. Almost everyone here is in the Church of Latter-day Saints."

"In the what?" I asked.

"The Church of Latter-day Saints—LDS. That's what the Mormons call themselves."

"Sounds like LSD," I giggled.

"Yeah, but it's definitely not."

"I was gonna sell my old junky furniture at a garage sale, but maybe I'll hang onto it, so you'll have something to start with." She had already concluded I would get the job and move to Utah, which made me feel good even if it was wildly improbable.

"Nancy, I appreciate your confidence, but what makes you so sure I'll get the job?"

She laughed. "These old farts would rather sit in their offices, looking important, than do any work. That's why they created these internships."

"Okay, now tell me what you really think."

"No, really," she said. "The only way they could get anybody to do so much shit work for so little money is to call it an internship." That's what I liked about Nancy—she didn't pull a punch.

❖

Josie and Dusty saw me off, waving good luck. West across Nevada, the long straight roads bisected the desert, country music on the radio. Even though in early September the worst of the summer heat had passed, a dry hot wind still blasted through the open windows—the little Peugeot had no air-conditioning. Not thinking much, watching the wide sky unroll from blue to silver, I turned off the radio to listen to the quiet of the desert-pulsing heat.

North past the Great Salt Lake, I drove east through the mountains, past Brigham City and Hyrum and down into Cache Valley. Logan was tucked between the Wasatch Mountains. It was like entering a dream. In late summer, the heat was tempered by the high elevation. The deep azure sky gleamed. I drove over the mountain pass, the valley spread out before me, the silver line of the Logan River snaking through the irrigated green alfalfa pastures. Where the fields weren't irrigated, dry soft golden brown rye grass waved in the breeze. Everything glowed with a clear mountain light. The last snow had melted off the highest mountains, and the gray cliffs and rock faces were solid in the clean air. After a couple of months of Los Angeles smog, this was heaven. It called to me. It felt right.

I passed groups of Hereford cows grazing in fenced pastures, spotted Appaloosa horses in makeshift corrals, silos of dairies in the distance. On the right side of the road, I noticed the first Utah State University sign, next to a complex of low brick buildings and fenced-in pastures with sheep—the Utah State prize-winning purebred Suffolks, Dorsets and Rambouillets. In the center of town stood the Temple of the Church of Latter-day Saints, a gray stone castle-like building with two white spires, surrounded by a tightly groomed park, begonias blooming.

Nancy told me that in Utah towns, the roads are numbered in relationship to the Temple. Her house was at 2300 West, 1500 North—twenty-three blocks west and fifteen blocks north of the Temple. The house had rundown clapboard siding with peeling paint, but the mountain backdrop made up for the shabbiness. Nancy's old Ford pickup truck was parked in the dirt driveway. She ran out to meet me wearing cowboy boots, blue jeans, a red bandana around her neck and a big welcoming smile.

I got out of the car and stretched. Nancy gave me a solid hug. She held me by the shoulders, leaned back and looked me up and down.

"You look fantastic!" she beamed. Hot and sweaty, I didn't think so, but I grinned, so happy to finally arrive.

"Let's get you settled in. You have an early morning tomorrow," she said, grabbing my bag.

After a dinner of tacos, beans, and beer, she gave me the fashion consult I needed to dress for success in Logan. "You can't appear too butch," she told me, looking at my short hair and chewed nails. "These guys are used to women in skirts and high heels with big hair."

I had only brought work clothes, thinking any interview for a large animal job would involve working in the barns, but Nancy told me I would be expected to meet Dr. Nelson in his office, and maybe meet the dean too.

"So what have you got?" I asked, glad we were about the same size. She found a gray skirt that just covered my knees, a white blouse and some low heels that fit me.

"Take your jeans and coveralls in case they let you near the animals," she advised.

"You can dress me up, but you can't take me out," I said, knowing that no matter what I wore, fashionably feminine was a stretch.

❖

Nancy drove me to the university early the next morning. The building was plain utilitarian brick, the halls a dirty cream color, the floors scuffed linoleum. We headed down a long hall. Nancy waved to the receptionist. She knocked lightly on the half-open door of Dr. Nelson's office and walked in, me trailing behind. Dr. Nelson's old wooden desk chair creaked when he stood up.

"Dr. Nelson," she said, "nice to see you again. I brought Dr. Rhodes over for her interview."

"Pleased to meet you," he said, coming around his desk and giving me a firm handshake.

"I'll leave you to it," Nancy said, brightly. She turned to leave, gave me a wink and closed the door. Dr. Nelson gestured to the metal chair in front of his desk. I took a seat.

He smiled a friendly smile and relaxed back into his creaky chair. He had light blond hair, piercing blue eyes, and pale, sunburned skin. I could picture his wife pressing the crease in his chinos. He looked at me quizzically as if he was trying to figure out what planet I had come from.

"Are you married?" First things first. I didn't wear a wedding ring, so he had to ask.

"Yes."

"Oh, wonderful" he exclaimed. "Did he come out here with you?"

"Actually, no, he's pretty busy."

"What does your husband do?"

"He's a musician."

"Oh really, what kind of music does he play?"

"Oh, lots of different kinds." I said, hoping that I could steer the conversation away from Vincent.

"Would he be willing to relocate if you came to Logan? You know the job is only for a year."

I didn't want to tell him that Vincent would probably figure I was joking if I told him I found a job in Utah, so I just mumbled something about how it wouldn't be a problem. Satisfied that he wouldn't be disrupting my marriage if he considered me for the job, Dr. Nelson proceeded.

"Let's take the truck and I'll show you around," he said, standing up. "The dean will meet us for lunch. He's interviewing all the candidates."

My heart sunk. All the candidates?

"How many candidates applied for the job?"

"Actually, we had quite a number of young men apply back in early spring." I thought of my application and wondered if he had forgotten that one young woman had also applied.

"Yes, but now that you have re-advertised the position?"

"Just you so far," Dr. Nelson admitted. He straightened some papers on his desk, not looking at me. "But we expect to have more since our new ad just went in JAVMA a few weeks ago." Good luck with that. I didn't know any new grads without jobs in August after graduation.

We drove by the dairy, the beef herd, the Sheep and Goat Institute, the Poisonous Plant Research Center, and finally, the Coyote Research Center several miles from campus, where the sheep ranchers funded research on coyote behavior to try and keep the varmints from eating their lambs. I was glad it was a driving tour because

I was wearing my feminine outfit, and my jeans and boots were back in Dr. Nelson's office.

The university sprawled over many acres. The campus felt sleepy. In late summer most students were gone. Dr. Nelson was more tour guide than interviewer. He asked no questions regarding my qualifications, skills, or experience. Weirder still, he said little about the job. Not a word about the hours, the responsibilities, the pay, the benefits. I figured we would get to that, maybe over lunch with the dean.

It was early afternoon when we walked through campus to meet the dean in the administration building. The dean's office was full of leather and bookshelves. Sunlight poured through a window with a view of the Wasatch Mountains. Dean Anderson was less a farm boy and more a polished administrator. He was tall and lean, a bit stooped, wearing a blazer, white shirt, blue tie, and loafers. His dark hair was slicked back, balding around the temples. He gave me a cool look and a weak handshake. "Nice to meet you," he said, and then turned to Dr. Nelson.

"Lamar, great to see you. Keeping busy?" he said, patting Dr. Nelson on the shoulder. "Why don't we proceed to lunch?"

I nodded and followed the two men across the courtyard to the faculty lunchroom. Heads turned when we sat down at a small round table with a linen tablecloth, cloth napkins and no coffee cups. No coffee was served. The end of the meal was signified by the men ordering large pieces of lemon cake. I leaned back in my chair and watched them eat. I was thinking of April and May in upstate New York, applying for jobs with the country vets. Wasn't a key part of the interview seeing the job applicant in action? Didn't they want to see how I could manage in the cow barn?

"I was wondering," I said, "after lunch, can we do rounds at the dairy? I brought my coveralls."

The dean looked at me a bit strangely and said, "My dear, are you really willing to get dirty?"

My face flushed, I clenched my fists under the table and said quietly, "Of course. I understand 'getting dirty' is a normal part of a large animal veterinarian's job."

I stared at the dean. Dr. Nelson signaled for the check. The room was full of men faculty chatting and finishing up their lunches, dishes were rattling in the kitchen, and all was right with the Utah State University world.

Getting dirty? Are you serious? I am a veterinarian, not a fashion model. I have been stepped on, drooled on, bled on, peed on, and shit on. I've held gobs of gooey placenta in my hands, had both arms up a cow giving birth, and had basketball-sized abscesses squirt pus all over me. Why the hell do you think I am here? Do you think I drove eight hundred miles at my own expense just for a tour of your university?

The waiter handed the check to Dr. Nelson, and the dean cleared his throat, now ready to get down to the business of the interview.

"Dr. Rhodes," he said in a solemn voice, "can you worm a horse?"

"Yes" I said, staring at him.

First, it was getting dirty. Now, we're going to have a list of all the run-of-the-mill stuff a large animal veterinarian does in the course of a day? Can you pull a calf, clean out a hoof, give a shot, dehorn a goat, treat mastitis, give intravenous calcium? No, it seems the dean was satisfied that knowing how to worm a horse was enough to qualify for the job. The dean's part of the interview was over.

We pushed our chairs back. The dean gave me a pat on the shoulder and said, "Nice of you to come by. Hope you have a good visit."

So you think I drove eight hundred miles to have a cozy little lunch with you?

Dr. Nelson walked me back to his office. He sat, leaning back in his creaky desk chair. I sat down in the chair in front of his desk, stiffly upright, a smile pasted on my face. He shuffled papers around on his desk. We looked at each other for a minute and then he stood, moving toward the door. I stayed put in my metal chair.

"Dr. Nelson," I said, "thanks for taking the time to interview me for the position."

"Happy to show you around," he said.

"I feel that I didn't get a chance to demonstrate my skills," I said, looking right at him. He looked away and reached for a bright red hard candy from the bowl on his desk. "We didn't talk about what you are looking for in a candidate."

He shifted from foot to foot, sucked on the candy, and looked down.

"Couldn't we take a few more minutes to talk about the job?"

"Linda," he sighed. "I would really like to spend some more time with you, but we've talked all morning, and I have an afternoon class I need to prepare for. I have your résumé with all your qualifications."

"Will you at least call me and let me know the results of your search?"

"Oh yes," he lied, "I'll call you in a couple of weeks."

❖

The next morning, Nancy and I went for breakfast at the Blue Bird Café, where we could get some coffee and decent eggs and potatoes. I said goodbye and hit the road for my eight hundred miles back to Altadena. Rolling through the desert, I thought about the magical nights in the redwood forests outside Mendocino, California, dancing to the Grateful Dead with my fellow commune dwellers under a yellow moon, falling down, laughing and spent, on the spring moss of the forest floor. Who would I have to be if I did get this job and move to Mormon land?

When I told the story to Josie and Dusty, they were suitably sympathetic. I still had a nagging hope. It was all demographics—I knew that in the whole country, it was unlikely that there were new grads available for that Utah job. Even if there were some around, they would assume that the job was filled by now, and the likelihood that they had seen the new ad was slim. The only way I knew about the job was from my trusty insider, Nancy. Although it was not logical, I thought about one other thing—the moment I drove over the mountains and dropped down into Cache Valley, I felt a magical connection. It was the right place for me.

Two weeks went by, it was late September, and I just couldn't stand it. I called. "Dr. Nelson!" I exclaimed cheerfully when he picked up.

"This is Dr. Rhodes calling. Remember? Dr. Rhodes, from California? I wanted to follow up about the internship."

Dr. Nelson sighed.

"Linda, I have been meaning to call you, but I've been so busy."

"Have you and the dean made a selection for the position yet?" I asked.

"Well, actually, we've been pretty frustrated."

"Really?" I said, trying to hold back and let him talk.

"We advertised in the vet journals, but no one applied." I waited. "But no luck, not even one new grad is available for the job." I kept my mouth shut, letting him talk.

"So . . ." he said slowly, "I have spoken to the Dean about how much work it is, and now that my teaching responsibilities have started, how much of a time commitment it is for me. He gave me the go-ahead to make my own decision." I could picture him shaking his head, running his hand through his hair, sitting back again in his creaky chair.

"I guess since you are the only applicant and because I'm desperate for help, I'll just have to give you a try."

There it was. My first large animal job offer.

"When can I start?" I asked.

PART TWO

Internship

CHAPTER 12

MY PARENTS BROKE OUT A bottle of champagne and Josie cooked Julia Child's special beef bourguignon recipe.

"So—Utah!" Dusty said, leaning back in his chair and mopping up the last of the gravy with a hunk of French bread. "There's some gorgeous country there—Canyon Lands, Arches."

"I'm glad you won't be three thousand miles away," Josie said.

"Did you call Vincent?" Dusty asked.

"Not yet," I said. "He's going to hate it."

"He should be happy for you!" Josie said.

All three of us took a sip of champagne at the same time. Josie set down her glass. We rarely talked about Vincent.

"Women follow men around for their careers all the time," I said. "I put up with living apart for four years, but now, if Vincent won't move, well . . ." I trailed off.

"He'll have to decide what's important," Dusty said. I nodded.

Josie cleared the plates, while Dusty went to the kitchen to make coffee. I sat back and sipped the last of the champagne, imagining Vincent and I with Spot, the cat, in a house near the Wasatch Mountains. Me with the job I'd been dreaming of and Vincent finding some musicians to play with, starting our life together. It could be good, couldn't it?

❖

For over a decade, Vincent was a fixture, an anchor in my life. Throughout relationships with other lovers, before and after our legal marriage, we had stayed connected. I clung to the thought that we would be together in some simulacrum of my parents' relationship once I finished vet school, and we could do what couples do. Sleep together each night, wake up to a routine that included love and support and stability. But my subconscious knew something was not right. I had dreams of trying to swim in my high school pool, but my strokes were futile, the pool was like Jell-O, almost solid, and try as I might to kick my feet and pull my arms forward, I was stuck, and I gave up trying to move, instead struggling to get out of the pool, the wet gel clinging to me.

Vincent never wanted to come with me to Philadelphia, and I never considered giving up vet school to be with him in Freeville. We kept our relationship, but it was hollowed out by that reality, and now here I was, again hoping that there was enough left between us to bear asking him again to follow me where I wanted to go, to give up his musical family and come with me as I pursued my dream job. I didn't realize I was ignoring the reality that was us, gelling around me. I didn't know how much we were operating on inertia, or perhaps my fear of loneliness, or his reluctance to hurt me, a bubbling mix of stuff that neither of us wanted to face. I didn't know it then, but it would take a catastrophe to wake us up and see that a relationship we had started when I was nineteen was no longer fit for purpose when I was thirty.

❖

Early in the afternoon I dialed the Freeville number. Vincent answered on the first ring, and I gave him the news, hoping at least he would be happy for me finally getting a large animal job.

"It's just a year," I said. "Not even, because the internship usually starts in May, so actually just nine months." Like so many phone calls between Vincent and me, silence prevailed. I held the phone, waiting.

"When do you have to start?"

"As soon as I can get there." I heard a deep sigh and imagined Vincent's sad brown eyes.

"Why don't you just come out and see the place? Cache Valley is beautiful, you'll love the mountains." I could almost hear his shoulders shrug. "Dusty said he would pay for your plane ticket to Altadena. Come to help me move, and we'll see how it goes."

"I can't come until next week," Vincent said. "We have a gig at Ithaca College."

That was the best I was going to get. No long discussion of the pros and cons, what the future might look like, how long he would agree to stay, what might happen when the internship was done. A week later, he was in Altadena. I gave notice to Dr. Jacobs. Josie and Dusty made me a surprise gift of the old green Peugeot.

❖

Spot had been in the hospital for over a month. He was a big boy, with long white fur spotted with calico, piercing golden eyes, and an industrial purr. After regular meals, flea baths, and love, he blossomed into a magnificent cat. When Vincent came to visit him at the vet hospital, Spot planted himself in the middle of the treatment room. When he saw me, he stood up, arched his back, and stretched. He stared at Vincent and walked directly to him, leaned his large body against Vincent's leg, and purred his loudest purr. Vincent bent down to pet him, and Spot rubbed his face against Vincent's hand.

Vincent smiled. "He's a handsome guy."

Retrieving the blanket from his cage, I said, "Come on, Spot," and scooped him into my arms. "You are coming home with us." I stroked his big head, and he closed his eyes. "Your new name is Logan, in honor of our first home together, in Logan, Utah." Logan was fine with that, and he settled into my arms, purring.

Packing was easy—my possessions were few. Dusty stood by the front door, his arm around Josie's shoulder. The sun was up, and lemon fragrance filled the air. I looked around at the house and garden, the live oak tree with its small dry leaves clinging to gnarled branches. It had been a good few months here.

Vincent was groggy—he hadn't slept well. I hoped we could make the long ten-hour drive in one day.

"Call us when you get there," Josie said. They were trying to be cheerful. I hugged each of them, knowing how much we would miss each other.

"You'll come and visit," I said firmly, hoping it was true.

"Sure," Josie nodded. Her hair grayed over the last year, the wrinkles around her eyes deepened.

Logan wailed a meow from his cat carrier. I hoped he wouldn't drive us crazy on the long trip.

"I'll drive," I said. Vincent climbed into the passenger seat, and everyone waved. As we drove down the driveway Vincent reached in the back, grabbed a pillow, set it against the door and closed his eyes. I drove through the Los Angeles traffic, Vincent fast asleep, and thought about what I was getting myself into, a challenging job in a Mormon world where my boss had already told me the only reason I got the job was because he was desperate.

We took turns driving, through Nevada and into Utah. Late at night we turned north and dropped down into Cache Valley. Logan was fast asleep on the back seat, exhausted from too much meowing and frantic staring out the window.

"It's so beautiful, I wish you could see the descent into the valley in the daylight."

Vincent shrugged. "I just want dinner and a shower. And a bed."

The plan was to stay a few nights with Nancy, who, being a night person, was waiting up for us. Logan was thrilled to be liberated and made himself at home, jumping on Nancy's couch and tucking in his paws. We had arrived.

CHAPTER 13

THE NEXT MORNING WAS A crisp October blue sky, mountain air Sunday. We woke up late to coffee, scrambled eggs, and fried potatoes. Vincent wandered outside to have a look at the mountains.

Nancy told me that Dr. Nelson expected me at work Monday morning at seven thirty a.m.—she would show me where to go. We could stay at her place for a few weeks while we looked for a rental. Nancy had her eye on a small stone house for rent. It was dilapidated, but she thought I would like it because it was at the end of a road, nestled up against the mountains.

Vincent and I explored the small town, bought some bread and cat food, wandered around the university, drove down the wide main street past the Temple. Logan was lovely, nestled in the broad Cache Valley, named for the fact that hunters used to cache the skins of fox, beaver, and even bear along the Logan River. The town was surrounded by two mountain ranges, rising up on either side of the valley, running north to south. Between the mountains were canyons, stretching from the valley east toward Wyoming and west to the Utah desert. The southeast corner of Idaho was less than twenty miles north.

Logan had one wide main street, lined with a few stores, banks, and gas stations, along with an auto parts place. Black walnut and oak trees shaded the Temple square. The Bluebird Café, where Nancy and I had coffee when I came for my interview, was a small antique ice cream and candy parlor, with a few tables for light lunches, on the main street across from the Temple. A few miles outside of Logan were small towns, no more than a post office and a few dairy farms—Nibley, Smithfield, Hyrum, Paradise, each a farming community where Mormons had settled in the 1850s.

After a long, hot day of getting acquainted with the town, Vincent and I decided to relax and treat ourselves to a beer. We parked the Peugeot and walked down the main street.

"Only one bar in town," I said. I couldn't remember the location, but we wandered around the side streets until we found it—windows painted over and a neon Budweiser sign in the window. It was a weekday. The bar was closed.

"We can buy a six-pack," Vincent said, but if there was a place to buy beer, it was well hidden. When we told Nancy about our search, she laughed.

"This is Mormon country! The only place you can buy beer is a state store. Come on, I'll drive you," she said, and we piled into her truck. She drove out to the edge of town where there was a prisonlike one-story cement-block building.

"This is the liquor store?" Vincent said, looking around at the few cars in the dirt parking lot.

"Yup. Highly regulated," Nancy said. "Look over there," and she pointed at a coal black pickup truck idling close by, with two young men inside.

"They just hang out and watch who comes and goes. Report folks to the bishop," Nancy said.

"And then what?" I asked.

"Then the bishop calls you, and you're in big trouble with the Church."

"What if you're not in the Church in the first place?" Vincent asked.

"They still keep an eye on you."

"A lot of people still drink," Nancy said. "They call them Jack Mormons—those who grew up in the Church, but drink alcohol and coffee and smoke too."

"I guess no one smokes weed," Vincent said.

"We keep very, very quiet about that," Nancy whispered, grinning.

I was charmed by the town. I wanted Vincent to be charmed too, but that was unlikely. There didn't seem to be a music scene here. Only one bar meant only one place for live music to be played. No guitar stores, either. Salt Lake City would have more live music, but it was two hours south. I watched Vincent, waiting for his reaction, but he kept to himself, not complaining, but not looking particularly happy either.

❖

As promised, Nancy drove with me early the next morning to the parking lot behind the Department of Animal, Dairy, and Veterinary Sciences building. Because I expected to be working, I wore a clean pair of jeans, a short-sleeved dark blue t-shirt, and work boots. Nancy pointed me to Dr. Nelson's office, then went to her old office to finish packing.

I sat waiting for Dr. Nelson and looked around. Typical state school—all metal furnishings, from the battered filing cabinets to the desk and dirty trash basket. A bowl of hard candy sat on Dr. Nelson's desk, a torn leather cushion on the desk chair, piles of paper and books on every surface, and a *Hoard's Dairyman* calendar from 1977 with a picture of a Guernsey cow on the wall.

I heard brisk steps coming down the hall, and Dr. Nelson walked in. Smiling, he shook my hand, pumping my arm up and down.

"How was your trip?" Dr. Nelson took off his baseball cap and smoothed back his hair.

"Fine," I said, smiling. I sat in the metal chair, and he leaned back, his desk chair squeaking under him.

"Are you settled in? Where are you staying?"

"We're staying with Dr. Hilber until we can find a rental."

I needed the "we"—a signal that my husband and I were together, that I was "normal," not some weird twisted single spinster.

"So, what does your husband plan on doing while you're here?"

"We're not sure, but he'll be looking for a job once we get settled." Dr. Nelson sat at his desk, opened his appointment calendar, and checked his "to-do" list.

I sized up Dr. Nelson as we chatted. He had a cheerful smile and a nervous chuckle. About six feet tall, trim, with strong arms and hands and a shy manner, almost self-deprecating. A hint of mischievous humor when he talked contrasted with the serious and restrained conversation of his fellow university Mormon friends. Over time, I learned that he carried a heavy workload—classroom teaching, university paperwork, Church duties, and family chores. He had four children, a small family by Mormon standards.

He walked me around the department and introduced me to my new colleagues, all men. I was an item of curiosity. The only woman in the vicinity was a secretary who looked up when I passed and frowned. The extension veterinarian, Dr. Clem Marten, a handsome, fit man with deep brown eyes, gave me a sincere, if rather bemused, welcome.

Dr. Nelson showed me my desk, a government-issue ugly metal thing with an equally ugly and uncomfortable metal chair, in a bare office painted gunmetal gray.

"Here's the locker room where we change," he said, pointing to a door. When I stepped forward to enter, he laughed nervously and said, "Dr. Rhodes, wait. That is the MEN's locker room."

There was no "MEN's" sign to be seen.

"Okay, sorry. Where's the WOMEN's?" A long moment of silence.

"Well, that's a problem." Dr. Nelson looked down at the floor and said, "Actually, we don't have one."

A woman who needed to change clothes had never worked here. I tried to imagine what I would do when I came back from farm calls covered in rotten placenta fluid, needing to change out of my smelly coveralls and wash off the slime. I didn't think the tiny sink in the ladies' room would suffice.

CHAPTER 14

WE DIDN'T TALK ABOUT HOW long Vincent planned to stay in Utah. He looked at rentals the first week while I was at work but hadn't come across anything better than the stone house Nancy had found. The house had been empty for a couple of months, so the landlord was happy to have us move right in, and the rent was cheap. It felt good to sign my name on the lease.

The small house was up against the foothills of the Wasatch Mountains, on the northeast side of Logan, the last house before the road turned to dirt and dead-ended in a gravel quarry. It was about four miles from the Temple, across the big irrigation ditch lined with peach leaf willow trees, that ran east–west, and brought fresh mountain melt water to the local alfalfa fields. Northern white cedar and Scotch pine trees decorated the surrounding hills and gave the air a wonderful oxygen-rich smell.

The house was different from most Logan houses, older, made from stone rather than wood. How old, I never found out, but likely from when the valley was first settled. It was set about two hundred yards off the road, in a scruffy field of goldenrod and milkweed. The trees in the front yard included a couple of tall oaks shading the house on either side. A long dirt driveway led downhill through a horse pasture.

I put down a box of books and stared out the large window in the living room that framed the mountains and the rangy front yard.

"There's no fireplace," I said, disappointed. I looked at the stained linoleum, a dark reddish color curling up at the edges of the floor.

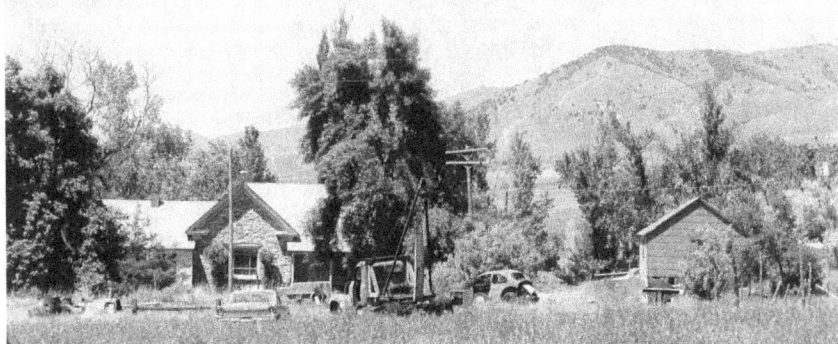

Stone house in Logan, Utah.

"But there is a chimney for a woodstove," Vincent said, bending down to peer into a drafty hole in the wall with a black metal pipe sticking out into the living room.

The nights were already cold that fall. I bought a small cast-iron woodstove to supplement the heat of the ancient oil furnace that forced tepid air through heavy iron vents in the floor. As I watched Vincent install the stove, I wondered if he could make this his home too. After a dinner of brown rice and stir-fried zucchini and tomatoes, we sat on the porch, watched the sun go down, and felt the chill mountain air. I watched Logan pouncing on acorns.

"Frank called while you were at work," Vincent said. Frank was Vincent's middle brother, a talented fiddle player.

"How's he doing?"

"Okay," Vincent said. I looked over at him. His eyes were dark and downcast.

"Something the matter?"

"He wanted to know when I'm coming back."

I knew we needed this conversation, but I didn't want to have it. The sky was dark blue. A bright fingernail moon hung just above the horizon, wispy clouds gray with the end of the sunset floating above. Logan leaned against my leg and purred. I patted his head.

"What did you tell him?"

Vincent reached over to pet Logan. "I told him I thought I'd stick around for a while and see how it goes."

I scooted over and put my arms around him, our faces close. "Really?" He smiled and leaned in to kiss my forehead.

We settled in. The best part of the house was the view of the Wasatch Mountains, receding in wilder and wilder layers into the distance. In winter, they were blanketed in the legendary powder snow of Utah, while in summer, thistle, cheat grass, and blackberry vines covered their steep sides, with cedar and juniper perfuming the air. On clear nights you could drive up to the gravel pit and watch the sunset across Cache Valley. Nothing separated us from the wilderness.

Frank sent some of Vincent's Freeville things—another guitar, some winter clothes. My books fit on the shelves, and the wood-stove gave off comforting warmth. Logan loved the outdoors, full of mice and chipmunks, safely far from traffic. In its old ugliness, the little house felt lived in, and I was determined to make it a home. For Vincent, I suspected only Freeville was home, but for now he seemed okay with the arrangement. We didn't talk about what might happen when I completed my internship.

❖

Logan was a solidly Mormon town, anchored by the Temple, built in 1884, only about thirty years after Brigham Young arrived in the Great Salt Lake valley. It was a university town with a small but exuberant non-Mormon counterculture. Vincent and I connected with a dozen or so ex-students, odd-jobbing for spending money, crashing on each other's couches, smoking dope, hiking, and skiing the canyons. Cache Valley was such a beautiful place that once they graduated USU, some decided to hang around, maybe for six months, maybe for a couple of years. A few of them had jobs at the university, some worked winters at ski resorts, others washed dishes in restaurants.

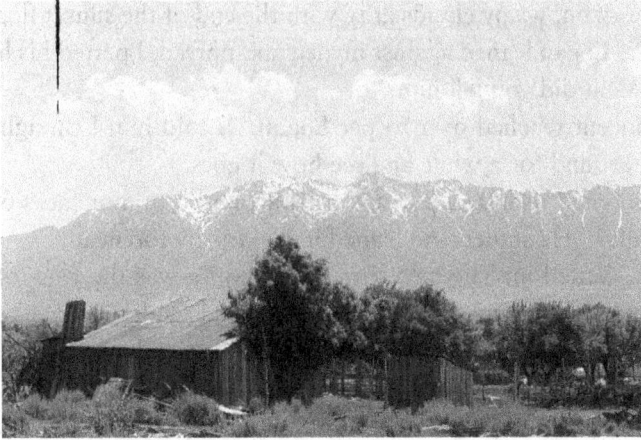

The backyard to the stone house in Logan with
the Wasatch Mountains in the background.

The Straw Ibis café was half a mile west of the Temple. The little shop served coffee and had floor-to-ceiling shelves stocked with merchandise, much of it handmade, plus an odd assortment of groceries. I was delighted to find open bins of lentils and almonds, organic whole wheat flour, hand-knit winter hats, and locally roasted coffee beans. Clearly no practicing Mormon would set foot in the Straw Ibis. Once we found it, Vincent and I went there not only to buy a few things but also to bask in the pseudo–northern California hippie vibe of the place. The bulletin board at the front of the store was crowded with handwritten notices about local poetry readings, pottery classes, and lost cats. Vincent paid for a pound of coffee and an organic chocolate bar while I perused the overlapping fliers.

"Here's someone looking for a guitar player," I said. He peered at the listing. *Local group looking for lead guitarist. Rehearsals on Sunday afternoon.* That was a coded message that the group was not going to services at the Temple on Sunday. Vincent tore off the little flap of paper with a phone number on it and tucked it in his jeans pocket.

The next time I was driving through town, I stopped at the Ibis for a cup of coffee. The woman ringing me up smiled. "You must be the new vet at USU," she said.

"How did you know?"

She looked me up and down and chuckled.

"I guess my outfit gave me away." I was wearing a stained pair of overalls, rubber boots, and a bandana tying my hair back.

"I'm Sally. I'm friends with Nancy. She told me about you." Sally came out from behind the counter. Her long, tightly curled hair was pulled into a bunch behind her head, her thick sweater was a lumpy knit-by-hand navy blue, her smile warm.

"You have a minute?" she said, motioning to a bench in the front of the shop. "We can chat."

The store was empty except for the two of us. I sipped my coffee, happy for the break. Sally asked me about Vincent, and I told her that her bulletin board had connected him with the local music scene. She told me her history. She was a third-generation Mormon from a prominent family, but she left the Church when she got married and opened a coffee-roasting business of all things. Her parents disowned her over it. Sally knew everyone in the Logan counterculture—they all shopped at the Ibis and hung out to plan cross-country skiing trips in the winter and tubing expeditions down the irrigation canal in the summer.

Vincent became the lead guitarist of a small group that played acoustic folk, jazz, and blues at parties up and down the canyon. The band never got paid much more than some booze or weed and maybe a few dollars, but they had a lot of fun. I was glad to see Vincent in his element. Even if they weren't his brothers, the musicians were good enough. I seldom had time to hang out with them. When I did, I couldn't get high because I was always on call, but at least I could enjoy the music and see a smile on Vincent's face.

CHAPTER 15

My job was to attend to the medical needs of the animals that belonged to the university. The Sheep and Goat Institute bred exotic ruminants like ibex and mountain goats, both species known for their spectacular horns. Just to the south of Logan was a large barn complex that housed the purebred, show-quality, blue-ribbon-winning sheep, which were used to teach sheep husbandry to the students. One block to the east of campus, a small working dairy milked about a hundred cows, raised heifers for replacement, and sold milk to the local dairy cooperative. Quite a menagerie.

"You getting settled?" Dr. Nelson asked a few days after I arrived. He glanced around my spare office. "Need anything?"

"I'm all set," I said.

Dr. Nelson perched himself on the corner of my desk. "Can't tell you how happy the missus is that I don't have to handle the late emergencies," he said. "I'm headed over to the bull stud to do some vaccinations. You want to come along?"

"What bull stud?" I didn't know Utah State kept bulls.

"It's not technically part of Utah State, but we provide their vet care, under a contract," he said. He stood, hitched up his pants, and smiled. "You're welcome to ride along."

"Can't this morning," I said. "I have to go over to the dean's office to fill out some paperwork for my benefits and stuff." I thought back on my job interview and the failed attempt to put a nose ring in a bull. I almost got myself killed. I hoped Dr. Nelson would take care of that part of the job.

My routine wasn't demanding. I arrived at the office at eight a.m. and checked the answering machine for any urgent requests—animals sick enough to need care right away. Most days there were no messages. I did routine care scheduled by the farm managers—foot trims, vaccinations, and blood tests. For the first few weeks, Dr. Nelson accompanied me on my rounds. I was glad for his experience and guidance.

My reception at Utah State University was chilly, at best. The farm managers were a bunch of crusty old guys. They did not like this whole idea of a lady vet, from the East, no less, and even worse, not a Mormon. I lacked the lifetime farm experience they expected of their veterinarian, and they were sure I would cause more problems than I would solve. Craig, the manager at the university dairy, was one of the worst. He was a tall guy in his late thirties, gut hanging over his belt. His handshake was strong, but he wouldn't look me in the eye, and his accompanying broad grin was a bit too wide. I didn't trust Craig. He seemed to focus somewhere over my shoulder when we talked, emphasizing his disinterest in what I had to say. I was trouble, pure and simple, as I had a lot of what he considered unnecessary work-generating ideas of how to keep cows healthier.

Craig sat in the dusty dairy office, just off the milking parlor, reading the latest issue of *Hoard's Dairyman*. I knocked on the open door and stepped in. He looked up and frowned.

"Got a minute?" He shrugged. "Can you show me your system for keeping reproduction records on the herd?"

He opened his desk drawer, pulled out a ratty old spiral notebook and handed it to me. "I write the breeding dates here, plus what semen we used." I flipped through the handwritten pages.

"And the medical records?"

He shrugged and pointed to his temple. "I keep those in here," he said. "I know my cows."

When I got back to the office, I wrote a memo, the first memo of my career. It outlined a plan to keep individual records for each cow on index cards, filed by number. While I was at it, I wrote up a schedule for preventive calf care and a plan to train the milkers in

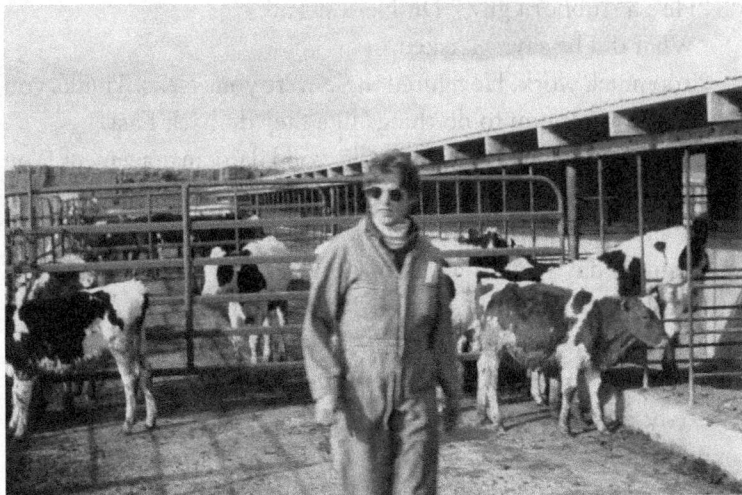

Linda walking the heifer pens at a Utah dairy.

better hygiene so the cows would get fewer infections. We needed to explain to the staff that if they didn't properly wash the cow's udders or keep the milking parlor clean, bacteria could migrate up the teat, causing mastitis, the infection of the udder I first saw in Irma the goat back on the California commune.

"Dr. Nelson, can I get your opinion?" I said, standing in his office door. I handed him the memo.

"What's this?" he asked.

"I had some ideas of how we could help make things easier at the dairy," I said. "I think it might be better if the suggestions came from both of us."

Dr. Nelson grinned. "All great ideas. Glad you tackled it." He pulled his glasses down over his nose and scanned the paper. He came out from behind his desk and shrugged his jacket on. "Why don't you let me read this over, and I can handle it with Craig?"

The next week, Dr. Nelson came into my office and handed me back my memo.

"He's a stubborn guy," Dr. Nelson said.

"What did he say?" I asked.

"Too much work. He figured these were your ideas. Thinks you are trying to get him to do things like they do back East."

"This isn't a 'back East' thing—its good dairy management. You know that, Dr. Nelson."

He sighed. "Craig wants to do things his way."

The next day I had to tend to a lame cow at the dairy, and as I walked by the dairy office, I heard Craig on the phone.

"Yup, that lady vet comes in here with all her new ideas from that eastern vet school, but she's never milked a cow in her life. We've been doing just fine up 'til now, thank you very much."

But I had milked cows. He had never bothered to ask. Craig was sure that if he waited me out, I would lose steam and give up. In less than a year I would be gone anyway, and he would have a new intern to irritate him.

CHAPTER 16

"DR. RHODES, WE GOT A cow down here looking pretty rough." It was Craig. He still wasn't convinced I was a real vet, even though I'd been on the job for a couple of months.

"What's going on?"

"She's not eating, and her milk is way off."

"How long has she been like this?" I asked, not expecting an accurate answer. Craig, I had learned, didn't pay close enough attention to the cows. They weren't his cows; they were the university's cows. Unlike most dairymen, he drew a salary. His income did not depend on whether the cows were healthy or sick, producing enough milk or not.

"Just noticed her this morning. Can you come down and have a look?"

A cow with no appetite gives significantly less milk, and making milk is her job. Dairy farmers measure milk in pounds. These girls can go from making a respectable eighty pounds of milk a day to ten pounds or less if they stop eating. Remembering that "a pint is a pound the world around" and that there are eight pints to the gallon makes the math easy—a cow with good production can give ten gallons of milk a day.

Dr. Nelson had told Craig if a cow was "off feed" that he should give her a couple of pink rumen boluses each day. These boluses, the term used for pills that are given to large animals, are big—about three inches long and an inch wide—and the shocking pink color of Pepto-Bismol, each one equivalent to a pint of milk of magnesia. They do virtually nothing for cows, but they make the farmers feel like they are helping. When I arrived at the barn, Craig was waiting for me and walked me down the row of cows to the one he was worried about.

The cardboard box that held twenty-four rumen boluses was sitting on a nearby shelf, half empty. I looked at the box, and then at Craig. Clearly, he had been treating this cow for a while.

I stood back and looked at my patient. She was a Holstein, mostly white with a few black patches over her back, weighing around a thousand pounds. Unlike the other cows digging into the fragrant fresh silage and hay, her head drooped, and her large brown eyes were dull. She turned her head when I approached, and I saw her big nose was dry—she hadn't been drinking enough. I walked around to examine her from both sides and the back and saw her abdomen was distended low over her left side. This made me suspect a certain diagnosis, but I didn't want to jump to conclusions. Being "off feed" and decreased milk production could be caused by dozens of things—the start of a respiratory infection, a viral infection of the gut, eating something she shouldn't have, like a nail inadvertently dropped in the hay (called "hardware disease"). But her ballooned belly made me suspect something different.

I stuck my thermometer in her rectum—it read 101.5 degrees, normal for a cow. Using my stethoscope, I listened in her left upper flank for the sound of a healthy rumen, a cow's first of four stomachs that should rumble with a contraction a couple of times a minute. All I heard was silence.

Craig was getting impatient.

"Come on, Doc, what do you think? Shall we give her some mineral oil?"

Keeping my hand on her side, I didn't look up.

"What about worms? These girls have been out on pasture all summer. Maybe she got missed when we wormed the herd a few weeks ago."

"Hmph," I grunted at him, trying to listen to the slow rhythmic beat of the cow's heart through my stethoscope.

"Maybe we should give her a big shot of penicillin."

"Hold on, Craig. I like to get to the diagnosis before starting treatment. Just let me finish this physical," I put my fingers to my lips to shush him while I listened to her lungs.

"Doc, I gotta get home to supper. Can't you speed it up?"

I pulled on a plastic sleeve covering my left arm up to my shoulder and inserted my arm into the cow's rectum to check her stool and palpate her uterus and ovaries. Her reproductive tract was normal. She would be ready to breed again soon.

"Did you change feed recently? Start a new batch of hay? Any of the other girls off feed?" I asked.

Craig shook his head no. The negative answer was consistent with my suspicion. I knew what was wrong with this cow. One final procedure would confirm my diagnosis.

I stepped to the left side of the cow and leaned against her warm bulk. The top of her back was at the level of my shoulders. I placed my stethoscope halfway down her bulging belly and gave her side a hard thwack by releasing my forefinger from my thumb. I heard a clear, distinctive ping. I did it again just for fun. "Ping!"

That sound indicates a left displaced abomasum, which vets call LDA and farmers call "twisted stomach." When the abomasum, the cow's fourth stomach, twists into this abnormal position, it fills up with gas, resulting in the ping sound when you smack the cow's side over the gas balloon. Hearing the "ping" is diagnostic and removes all ambiguity in treatment—the cow needs surgery. An LDA gives the cow a hell of a bellyache, so she stops eating. Once corrected, in most cases she will be back to normal in a week or so.

Straightening up, I said confidently, "She has a twisted stomach—a left displaced abomasum." Craig looked at me, eyebrows arched, his blue eyes blank.

"I'll have to schedule surgery, but it's not an emergency." I patted the cow's rump and dropped the manure-stained plastic sleeve in the trashcan. "I can do it tomorrow."

"Our cows don't get that," Craig said.

This did not register with me, so I kept chatting, showing off my knowledge, about how it was probably caused by low calcium after she'd calved a couple of months ago plus the recent addition of some corn silage to the feed.

He said a little louder, "Our cows don't get that." Now he had my attention.

"We've never had a twisted stomach in this herd," he said, his voice deep, his chest out. He was right and I was wrong.

"I've never seen one, and I've been working on dairies my whole life."

I squatted down next to the tackle box, putting away my stethoscope and thermometer, smiling. I knew what I knew.

"You just think she has a twisted stomach because that is what the cows get out East."

Craig was right in one sense—we did see a lot of LDAs in the East. No one knew precisely why, probably related to diet. In Utah, where cows were fed lush, high-quality alfalfa hay, LDAs were rare. But rare doesn't mean never. The cow standing here had an LDA, and the only treatment was surgery. No matter how many pink rumen boluses Craig shoved down her throat, her stomach was not going to untwist on its own.

"You aren't doing surgery on my best cow, Doc! That's crazy." Now this old white cow was suddenly his best cow.

"We've never had a surgery like that here. I won't permit it." Pulling rank on me—that was interesting. I stopped fiddling with my tackle box and stood up. Craig puffed out his chest like a rooster, arms crossed, feet wide, glaring down at me. He was a good six feet in his sweaty socks. We looked warily at each other.

Although the cows did not belong to him but to Utah State University, he was in charge of their care. I looked at the cow, and she looked at me. She was either having surgery, or she would go gradually downhill and end up slaughtered for meat. I walked over to the sick cow and leaned on her left side.

"Craig, come over here. See this bulge in her side? That's gas from the twisted stomach." I pointed to the large beach ball bulge.

"You can hear the gas in there. Listen." I handed him my stethoscope.

I thwacked the cow's side several times watching Craig's solemn studious frown. I thwacked her so hard I heard the ping without the stethoscope. With it, the ping must have been deafening. Watching him look so serious, stethoscope in his ears, I grinned. I was sure of what I knew; I enjoyed showing Craig that I could figure stuff out and help his cow.

He stood up and said, "She's just got some gas. I'll let her run around the pasture, and she'll pass it just fine." He stared at me, defiant. Although a run around the pasture might have a slim chance of untwisting the abomasum, it would be a minor miracle if it did. I pictured the cow gallivanting around the pasture, passing massive amounts of gas, and chuckled.

"Your call. You're the boss. But you know what, let's let Doc Nelson have a listen and see what he thinks. He and I will come down tomorrow morning after milking."

By the next morning, Doc Nelson and most of the veterinary staff, including the department chairman, had heard about my laughable misdiagnosis of an LDA in a Utah cow. How could I be so foolish as to think a cow in Utah would ever have such a problem? Everyone knew that the high incidence of LDAs in the East was because those farmers didn't know how to feed cows properly. There was a lot of headshaking and remarking on my inexperience.

Doc Nelson met me at the barn. The cow was standing up, not eating, looking thin and hunched—a cow with a bellyache. Doc Nelson did his version of a physical exam. He was rushed, a little less thorough than me, but he noticed the same lack of rumen movement I had heard. When he did the rectal exam, he felt the same things I'd felt. I watched him carefully, waiting for him to get to the "pinging" part of the physical, but he just stood up and said, "Can't find much wrong with her. Let's just start her on some antibiotics. Maybe she has a bit of a gut infection."

I realized he had absolutely no idea how to "ping" a cow. No wonder there were no LDAs in Utah—probably none of the vets had been taught how to diagnose the condition. I pretended he had just missed it.

"Doc Nelson, I hear it best when I put my stethoscope right here," and then I thwacked that cow for all I was worth, so hard she jumped. I figured he could hear the ping from five feet away. He looked thoughtful, probably wondering what the heck I was doing.

He said, "Are you absolutely sure she has an LDA?"

"The ping is clear as a bell," I said, still not sure he knew what a "ping" was.

He cocked his head to one side and raised his bushy blond eyebrows. "If you say so, you should do the surgery, but I want to be here to see it."

He was giving that crazy lady cow vet just enough rope to hang herself. I gave him a short nod. "I'll get my instruments sterilized and meet you back here before the afternoon milking, say three o'clock?"

"Fine. We better get her out on the pasture where it's cleaner," he said. Good idea. Doing surgery in the barn would be hard—too crowded, dirty, and not enough light.

"Craig, can you get this old girl out back by three this afternoon? Get her on some clean grass?" Craig nodded, not looking at me. Dr. Nelson was his boss.

❖

It was settled. The lady cow vet would do LDA surgery at Utah State, the twisted stomach would be nowhere in evidence, and everyone would have a good laugh and a good story to tell. No harm done.

Even though I was as certain of this diagnosis as I was that my patient was a cow, I was nervous. I'd never done an LDA surgery by myself.

I pulled out my surgery textbook and reviewed the various surgical approaches—left flank in a standing cow, dorsal recumbency, and midline—and the details of the procedure. I had assisted on dozens of LDA surgeries as a student, but this would be the first where I was the chief (and only) surgeon. Doc Nelson would be there if I needed help, which was somewhat of a comfort, even though he had no experience in this procedure.

I tried to eat lunch, but my sandwich was too dry in my mouth. I gulped some instant coffee secretly in my office, but that made my nerves worse.

The day was perfect—a clear blue sky, cottonwood trees in the valley turning yellow and gold, October sunshine haze in the air. When I pulled up to the dairy, pickup trucks were lined up, parked along the driveway, like folks were arriving for a barn sale. I walked around the back of the barn, looking for my patient. What I found was an impromptu theater-in-the-round.

The cowboys had set up an amphitheater made of hay bales, with several tiers of seats surrounding the star of the event, the big white cow. They were talking and laughing but fell silent when I walked around the barn. It took a minute for it to register that this was my audience. They had come to see the lady cow vet do surgery.

Doc Nelson walked up. "Hope you don't mind," he said, waving to the peanut gallery. "Some of the boys thought they could learn something. They've never seen an LDA before." He smiled sheepishly.

We both knew they weren't there to learn anything. Craig was nowhere in sight. I guess he was so sure I was crazy that he didn't even bother showing up. The cow was standing quietly, tethered by a halter to the fence. I drew up a dose of tranquilizer and injected it into her jugular vein. The group ignored me. I could hear a low buzz of chat about the weather and the hay crop.

I ran an extension cord from the barn, fired up the large clippers and began shaving the thick hair off a good portion of the cow's left side, where the incision would be. This was prickly work—cow hair is coarse, and the clippers threw out sharp little bits of bristle that stuck to my sweaty face and arms. The loud clipper buzz mingled with the drone of the cicadas in the tall grass around the barn.

I dragged the hot water bucket close to the cow and washed her left side. I'd decided on the left flank approach. The warm sun made me sweat under my coveralls. My hair was tied back with a bandana, so I wouldn't make the mistake of breaking sterility by pushing hair out of my eyes.

Doc Nelson wandered over, all relaxed and smiling.

"Can you give me a hand once I scrub up and help me open up the sterile stuff?"

"Sure," he grinned. "Just tell me where you want everything."

I swabbed my patient's left flank with an antiseptic solution and began to scrub her newly naked skin with a small brush. "I'll set up on that hay bale over there. Just put this clean towel down, will you?"

Not used to the role of chief surgeon, I felt weird directing my boss, but he was clearly ceding control. If someone was going to look foolish here, it was not going to be him.

The cow was standing quietly—the tranquilizer helped. I numbed her up with a lidocaine injection so she wouldn't feel the incision. She would stand throughout the procedure, with me on her left side. She might not like me mucking around inside her, putting her stomach back where it belonged, but I hoped she would stay calm, She would feel much better once that gas was out of her constricted abomasum. The cowboys quieted down and took their seats. The feature show was about to begin.

There's nothing more solemn than a surgeon putting on gown and gloves. It looks just like on TV, except I was standing in a cow pasture. I didn't wear a mask because it seemed kind of silly for a procedure being done outside, complete with flies and dust in the air.

The cowboys were leaning forward, elbows on knees, waiting for the big moment. With a large scalpel, I made an eighteen-inch-long cut through the skin of the flank, neatly going deep enough to cut through the skin but not deep enough to penetrate the muscles. Several small but vigorous bleeders began to squirt bright red blood over my surgical gown as the skin fell open to reveal the pale tissue beneath.

If the cow had an LDA, once I cut through the flank muscles and into the abdominal cavity, the bright pink, shiny abomasum would bulge through the opening, and I would be proved right. If all we saw was the top of the rumen, I would be proved wrong, stitch her up and admit defeat. The audience probably had no idea of what they might see next, but the vision of the lady cow vet doing surgery was entertaining on its own.

I extended the incision through the flank muscles and immediately knew my diagnosis was correct because I could see the balloon of the abomasum. There it was, a thing of beauty—the pink, gaseous displaced abomasum. Doc Nelson looked over my shoulder, nodded, and stood back. I pushed the distended stomach down and forward, where it belonged, reaching into the cow's belly up to my armpit. The abomasum lurched back into place and made a gurgle of gas as it deflated. The poor cow gave a huge sigh—we both felt a whole lot better. I stitched the abomasum in place so it wouldn't twist again.

"Well, doggone it, that is the first LDA I have seen around these parts," Doc Nelson said. "Can't think of why she got it. You reckon it's the new silage we're feeding?"

I nodded again. Bad silage was often implicated in LDAs. "Think we ought to check calcium levels on the fresh cows?" Dr. Nelson was chatting away, intrigued at this medical mystery, and not at all disappointed that I was right. It felt good to be having a doctor-to-doctor conversation. He was asking my opinion.

"Good idea," I said. "Low calcium can contribute to the condition."

Sewing up the skin, I was concentrating so hard I didn't notice my audience had up and left. The show was over. I stood back and looked at the neat line of sutures, dark brown surgeon's knots of catgut holding the thick skin together, not too much tension, skin just opposed, to allow for better healing. Pulling off my bandana, I shook out my hair and leaned against the fence, feeling the afternoon breeze cooling down, wafting the sharp smell of cow manure and silage.

The old cow was a bit wobbly, not surprising considering what she had been through. I gave her an injection of penicillin and walked her back to the hospital stall, where she promptly lay down with a grunt. Doc Nelson put his hands on his hips, tilted his head, and gave me a little wink.

"Well, I guess you showed us, little lady!"

CHAPTER 17

IN THE FIRST MONTHS OF my internship, I did routine stuff, probably what Dr. Nelson thought the girl vet could manage. Occasionally, I got kicked and sported a nasty bruise for a week or so. Getting dirty was part of the job, and I didn't mind unless it got extreme. One afternoon, as I stepped up to give an injection, the cow let fly with a huge pee, and I got a stinky soak. After a hot shower and a change of clothes, I was fine. This was part of being a large animal vet, and as long as my patients got better, I was happy.

Most days I didn't have enough work to keep me busy. On slow days, Dr. Nelson and I went to the dairy barn to practice pregnancy checks. I was gradually getting the hang of palpating the cows' uterus and ovaries. I was determined. I remembered that snotty California vet bragging about how good he was at rectals, and I knew with enough practice I could do a hundred rectals in a day too. Maybe next year I could go back and apply for that job and show him what a determined woman could do.

The slow pace of work grew boring as the year wore on. It was 95 percent routine and 5 percent crazy emergency. "Doc, come quick, we got a cow with her foot stuck in the cattle guard!" or "You know that cow that calved yesterday? She's out in the pasture and cast her withers," the lay term for a prolapsed uterus.

Emergencies got my heart pumping. In most cases, I had only a textbook idea of what to do or, if I was lucky, had seen the condition once in school. In other cases, the situation was unique. I needed to think on my feet and call on my knowledge of anatomy, good medical treatment, and correct drug dosages.

Struggling with my fear and anxiety by myself was hard. Not only was I the only woman veterinarian at the university, I suspected I was the only one in the entire state. One day, I called New Bolton Center at Penn to speak to Dr. Elaine Hammel. She had coached me through a couple of calvings when I was her student, and the way she remained calm during tough cases had impressed me.

"Dr. Hammel, it's Linda Rhodes. I rode on field service with you last year."

"Linda! How are you doing? Where are you?"

I explained about the search for a cow job and the Utah State internship.

"That's wonderful. Sounds like you're finally doing what you set out to do," she said, sounding pleased.

"At least it's a first step." The story of the failed New York job search and my concern over finding a job post-internship was too long to tell. "I'm calling to ask you a question. Some of these emergency calls, I get a bit panicky."

"Uh huh," she said. "I understand."

"What if I get to the farm and the situation is more than I can handle?"

"I know what you mean."

"How long before you get over that feeling? How much experience does it take to feel like you can handle it whatever the problem?"

I heard her quiet laugh. It made me remember how much I liked and respected this woman.

"You know, Linda, our work can be really challenging, and there have been many times in my career that I've been worried I won't be able to handle a situation." I pressed my ear to the phone, glad that I called her. "I'll let you in on a secret. You never stop being scared by those difficult cases. You just stop showing it."

My confidence grew in tiny increments, balanced by buckets of doubt. I hit that vein on the first try and gave the right antibiotics. The calf's fever was down the next day, and I went home glowing with pride. That little calf that had been coughing for a week and could hardly suckle it was so hard to breathe was gulping down her bottle, eyes bright.

The next day, I tried to carve out a foot abscess on a cow, and she kicked me into a pile of manure in the gutter. No matter how I tied her foot, she still managed to kick enough that I couldn't get the pus to drain. Maybe those naysayers were right. A woman just didn't have the strength for this. That night I couldn't sleep, full of doubt. By the morning, my determination back, I tackled that foot again, this time with a sedative that knocked the cow off her feet, and damn if I didn't get a pint of pus out of that foot. After an expert bandage job, she was up and walking, and I imagined how relieved she felt.

My confidence see-sawed, unbalanced, up and down in wild swings.

After the high drama of my first C-section, when the cow and calf both did fine, the balance steadied. There were still days when I confronted a challenge that sent me into the darkness of doubt, but they came less frequently. I was beginning to believe it just might be possible for me to be a good veterinarian.

❖

After lunch on an unseasonably warm fall day, I found a message on my desk. Craig had called about a fresh cow down with milk fever. It's a funny term because the condition has nothing to do with a fever; rather, it's caused by low blood calcium. I saw a lot of milk fever cows in the summer after my sophomore year in vet school that I spent riding ambulatory at Cornell. I remember Dr. Mary Smith standing next to a bulky black-and-white Holstein who had given birth a few days prior.

"Calcium is required for muscle activity. When a cow gives birth and her milk supply is at its peak, she's called a 'fresh' cow. If too much of her calcium goes into her milk, she collapses and can't get up because her muscles won't work." Dr. Smith fit the tubing on a bag of calcium solution. "The treatment is about half a liter of intravenous calcium." She stuck the needle into the cow's jugular vein in one smooth move and attached the tubing to the bag of calcium.

"Linda, get your stethoscope and listen for irregular heartbeats." I knelt next to the cow and listened to her heart as Dr. Smith started the flow of calcium.

"The heart is also a muscle, and it is particularly sensitive to calcium levels. Too much calcium, given too fast, can stop the heart cold. So, it's important to administer a calcium drip slowly and to monitor the heart rate. If the heart rate becomes irregular or the heart skips beats, stop the calcium drip for a few minutes until the heartbeat stabilizes."

I listened, the cow's big heart beat steady and strong, and just when the calcium bag emptied, she struggled to her feet and walked away as if nothing had happened.

"She'll be fine," Dr. Smith said. "Some farmers do their own IVs, but I would rather they call us. Calcium given too fast kills cows."

❖

I was planning an afternoon trip to the dairy to check on a calf I'd started on antibiotics a few days earlier, so I checked the truck to make sure I had a couple of bags of calcium and drove over. The dairy office was quiet. Flies buzzed in the corners of the sunny window when I peeked in. No sign of Craig. I collected my IV infusion set and the bag of calcium fluid and went looking for the down cow.

I found her sprawled in the alleyway where she had collapsed on her way back from the milking parlor. She was a huge cow, almost all white, with a patch of black on her rump. She didn't look too bad—her head was up, her forelegs tucked under her chest. When I lifted her tail and let it fall, it thwacked to the concrete floor, limp, a sure sign of milk fever. I slapped her rump and yelled at her to get up, and she looked at me with her sad brown eyes.

I wanted more of a history. When did she go down? How much milk is she producing? When had she delivered her calf? No one was around to ask, and Craig's medical records were all in his head. I wanted someone to listen to her heart through a stethoscope while I ran the calcium into her vein, like I had been taught was best practice. At least I could feel her pulse while the fluid was running, and that should be good enough. I stuck her jugular vein with the long stainless steel needle, hooked it up to the bag with the calcium fluid and started the drip, holding it awkwardly with one hand, bent over with my other hand on her neck, feeling her strong steady pulse.

The cow was still, her breath regular, the barn quiet. I held the drip low to slow the flow of calcium. Her pulse was steady. I sweated under my coveralls standing in the direct sun, and my mind wandered to the little calf I had to check when the cow made a strangled grunt and her pulse disappeared. I yanked the needle out of her neck, dropped to my knees and put my ear on her chest. Her heart had stopped without warning, and that grunt was her last gasp. There was nothing I could do.

Standing up, I felt tears prick my eyes. I stared at the dead cow, so still on the ground, her eyes wide open. So sudden, this death. Less than half a liter of calcium. She was a huge cow. A cow her size should take up to two liters. My stomach churned, nausea rising in my throat. Sweat dripped down my back. The concrete floor was cool under my knees. I sat back on my heels and covered my face with my dirty hands.

I had treated a dozen or so milk fever cows in Utah and many more when I was in school. In some of those cases, the skipped heartbeat alerted me to trouble, and I slowed or even stopped the calcium while the cow's heart stabilized. I thought I knew how to do this. But here was my patient dead at my feet, evidence that I was not so good at this after all.

I had to find Craig and let him know, so he could get the front loader and drag her carcass out for disposal. I gathered up the half-filled bag of calcium and the IV tubing and walked through the milking parlor. I tossed the fluid bag in the garbage can and headed to the truck but then stopped; something caught my eye. I went back to the garbage and took a closer look. Three IV bags were in the trash—the one I'd just tossed and two under it. Why were there two empty bags of calcium in the trash? It occurred to me that Craig had treated this cow with a couple of bags of calcium, and when she didn't get up, he called me. If I had known what he had done, I might not have given her that third bag. I felt even worse that I was trying to blame Craig for what was my mistake. Maybe if it was his fault I wouldn't feel so bad. How could I be sure those bags had been used on the cow I killed?

Craig was nowhere in sight. I was going to have to tell him I killed his cow. He would probably say it was his best cow too. I felt my eyes go puffy and my chest tighten, but I was determined not to cry.

❖

At the office, I found Dr. Nelson sitting at his desk.

"Treated a down cow at the dairy," I said. Dr. Nelson looked up, saw my face, and closed the door.

"Sit down, Linda."

"I must have run the calcium too fast, her heart stopped," I said, my face wet with tears. God, I hated to be the lady vet who cried.

"Happens to the best of us," he said, giving me a quick pat on the shoulder.

"Never happened to me before," I said. I took a deep breath. I could almost hear Doc Nelson thinking only girl vets cry.

"Didn't they tell you in school that if you haven't killed a cow with calcium, you haven't treated many milk fevers?"

As he said that, I did flash back to Dr. Hammell at Penn saying that very thing. I gave a half-hearted smile and nodded.

"So, what happened?" he asked. I told him, leaving out the part about the extra calcium bags in the trash and my suspicion that Craig had treated the cow himself before he called me.

"Did you talk to Craig yet?"

"Not yet. He wasn't around."

"I'll talk to him. Every time something like this happens, he claims it was his best cow," Dr. Nelson said, leaning back in his squeaky chair. "You don't need to hear that."

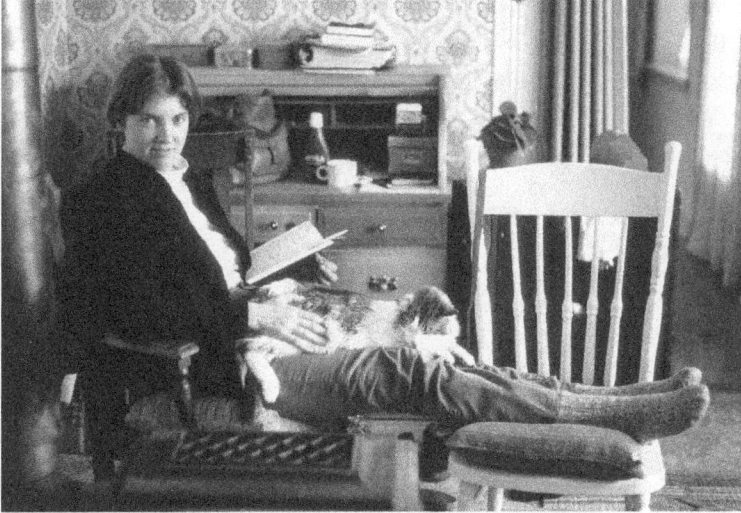

Linda and Logan at home in the stone house.

I dreaded seeing Craig, but knowing that Dr. Nelson didn't make a big deal out of it helped. Even so, I felt bad. Really bad. I went straight home, put on my hiking boots, and took the path up the mountain gully. I wanted to get high up, where I could get the long view. Once the sun dipped below the horizon, tinting the clouds a deep red, I walked home.

❖

"Where were you?" Vincent asked. I could see he had set the table, and something was cooking on the stove.

"Up the canyon," I said, pulling my boots off.

I sat on the old wooden chair next to my desk, the heat from the woodstove warming my feet, Logan on my lap, and sighed. I so needed consolation and reassurance. Vincent was sick of me talking about work, and work was all I wanted to talk about. I was never going to get this balance right.

"How was your day?" I asked.

CHAPTER 18

AFTER THE ATTEMPTED NOSE RING placement and my smashed leg on that ill-fated job interview, I was relieved that I didn't have to treat dairy bulls. Most dairies don't keep bulls. Instead, they breed their cows with artificial insemination. For a few months after they are born, the little bull calves are as cute and gentle as their sisters, and some can be trained to show by 4-H kids. But when they go through puberty, they become one of the most aggressive and dangerous domestic animals. They are humongous, muscular, powerful animals with wild eyes and the desire to crush you into dust.

The first year I was in Utah, the teenage son of one of the local dairymen went into a pen with the 4-H bull he had raised from a calf, shown to win several blue ribbons, and fed and watered daily. On this particular day, that bull butted him, knocked him down with his mighty head, pushed the young man up against the fence and crushed him to death, all in the space of a few minutes. Meanness is just part of the genetics of those high-testosterone bulls.

One such bull stud facility was in Logan, and Dr. Nelson was their veterinarian. An easy job, for the most part, because the bulls were looked after by an experienced and well-trained staff, fed optimal diets designed by veterinary nutritionists, and kept in air-conditioned pens that were cleaned regularly—conditions generally unavailable to ordinary, run-of-the-mill cattle. They were not allowed on pasture, because no normal pasture fence could hold them if they decided to run. Instead, each bull had a generous outdoor pen, enclosed by sturdy steel fencing.

The university contracted with the bull stud company to provide their veterinary care. Dr. Nelson visited the facility every now and then, hung out with the collection technicians, walked through the barns to have a look at his charges, and commented on how well things were going.

One late fall day, with a haze settled over Cache Valley, Dr. Nelson decided, since things were slow, that I should have a look at these amazing animals. We drove up in the vet truck and parked next to the low building. Jeb, the manager, came out to greet us.

"Doc!" he said, "How you been?"

As he was speaking to Dr. Nelson, he eyed me sideways, not acknowledging my presence. Jeb had deep-set eyes and the weathered skin of someone who worked outside. His high forehead sported a baseball cap with the black and green company logo on it, which also decorated his clean, pressed coveralls. I noticed a large gold wedding ring on his thick, callused left hand. He was easy in his body with the fitness you see in farmers, from real physical work, not workouts at a gym.

Doc Nelson said, "This is Dr. Rhodes, she's our intern this year. I thought she would get a kick out of seeing the boys."

Jeb's eyebrows went up to his hairline, and he reached out with a hand as big as a catcher's mitt for a firm shake. He ushered us into the cool building, the entryway displaying large glossy color pictures of bulls, all standing sideways and looking regal. We dipped our boots in neon blue disinfectant and went through a door to the lab, quiet and empty, freezers humming, microscopes covered. On the far end of the lab was another door, where we again dipped our boots and walked down a long hall to the barn area.

"Hay crop was good this year," Jeb said.

"Yup" Doc Nelson replied. "Second cutting coming in."

"What did you think of the Aggies basketball this year?" Jeb asked. All Utah State's sports teams were nicknamed the Aggies.

"Don't follow basketball much. I'm a baseball man," Doc Nelson said.

Jeb turned to me and said, "If you want to see a collection, you're in luck." He opened the far door, and I saw a long row of huge stalls running down the left side of the building. Muffled breathing and an occasional snort broke the quiet. The air was thick with the smell of manure, silage, and disinfectant.

"They'll stick their heads out soon enough to see who the strangers are," Jeb said, and sure enough, one by one, each Holstein bull's massive head appeared over the thick wooden door of the stall, staring in our direction. My first thought was *My God, they are huge*, followed quickly by *and dangerous*. They rolled their large eyes back in their heads and snorted. Tongues dripping saliva lolled out of their mouths, and one bellowed—a deep, resonant sound that echoed throughout the barn. They pawed the ground, banged and crashed against the steel reinforcements in their stalls, the racket signaling their aggression and dominance.

On the backside of each stall was a door that could be opened to the individual large outdoor concrete pens. At the far end of each outside pen was a shelter for shade and a water trough. I saw a worker on a small yellow front loader in one of the outside pens scrapping the impressive pile of manure a bull had produced.

We walked the length of the barn. Twenty massive heads swiveled to watch as we passed. White and black patches of curly hair covered their heads. They wore nose rings the size of large dog collars. An ineffable feeling of malevolence hung in the air, as if they were thinking, "I will kill her. Yes, I will. Just let me out," as they drooled and snorted.

Most places when I saw animals, even at zoos where I knew it would be dangerous, I had an urge to reach out and pet or at least touch them. Here, I had the urge to pull away, but I also felt an awe of this power and majesty, dominance and grandeur. Magnificent beasts.

Jeb said cheerfully, "These boys will kill you soon as look at you. They'll trot nice and easy down the alley to do their business, but we never turn our backs on them."

Jeb was matter-of-fact about the sex. He showed me the collection room, the mounts, and the banks of freezers. He opened one, and clouds of cold vapor from the liquid nitrogen rose up. Jeb pulled up a long aluminum rod, studded with small glass ampules of frozen semen, each neatly labeled with collection date and bull identification in tiny, black letters.

Jeb addressed his patter to Doc Nelson. I tagged along behind.

"So, Doc, how's the missus?"

"Working on the church social this Sunday," Doc Nelson said. "Baking, mostly. Kids driving her crazy."

"See you there," Jeb said. "My wife is doing the baked beans." He looked at me. "You want to stay to see a semen collection?"

"Sure, I'd love to." Dr. Nelson looked at his watch. "Guess we have time before lunch," he said. "I'm hoping to get over to Salt Lake for the rodeo tonight."

Two young men in coveralls were busy in the collection room, getting set up for the big event, warming the artificial vagina, a large latex tube, in a water bath, and readying the mount that looks like a gymnastics pommel horse and is meant to be a fake cow.

"Dr. Rhodes, you stand over here," Jeb said, indicating a corner of the room. "If the big guy sees you, it might distract him."

Grunting and making a deep-throated groaning sound, the bull came down the alleyway, one technician leading him with a rope through his nose ring, the other behind.

"He knows the drill," Jeb said. "They get excited just walking down the hall." The bull came into the collection room with a full erection, penis a yard long, bobbing up and down as he walked. He charged right at the mount and jumped on it, thrusting.

One technician grabbed the bull's penis while the other held the artificial vagina and directed the stream of ejaculate into a collection vessel. The bull slid off the mount, panting, his tongue lolling from his open mouth. It was all over in just a few minutes.

"That's all there is to it," Jeb said. "Most of the time, it's pretty easy."

"Most of the time?"

"Well, last week we had a situation. Bull came down the corridor fine, but something spooked him." We watched the tech pour the semen into a sterile beaker. "That sucker knocked over the mount and went at it like he wanted to kill it," he said, chuckling. "We hightailed it out of there until he calmed down."

Jeb took the beaker of semen into the lab and held it up. "I'll let it cool down. Looks like once we extend this, we'll get three or four hundred straws." That would be enough to fertilize that many cows.

"How often do you collect?" I asked.

"Depends on the bull. Some of my guys can go every day. We generally do three times a week."

Doc Nelson and I drove back up the hill to the university.

"Those big boys are seriously dangerous," Doc Nelson warned. "Jeb isn't kidding—they will kill you. Never get in the stall with them, even if they are tied up, without tranquilizing them."

I nodded.

"Just let the doggone bull die," Doc said. "Rather him than you."

"Did you ever have to treat any of them?"

"Once," he said. "Bull had a foot abscess. Jeb tied his head. I reached over and jabbed him with a big dose of tranquilizer. Once a bull goes down, you have about thirty minutes to complete the treatment and get out of the pen." He parked the truck and turned very serious. "And the bull wakes up with you on the right side of the fence. Never, ever turn your back on him!"

I nodded and prayed that I would never have to use his advice.

CHAPTER 19

"LINDA, COME ON IN HERE," Dr. Nelson hollered. He saw me walking by his office late in the day with my filthy coveralls, hair pulled back in a red bandana, stinking of cow manure after being called to look at a calf with diarrhea at the dairy barn.

He laughed. "You are a bit of a mess, young lady."

I pulled up the old wooden chair by his desk and sat down with a sigh. I'd been up since five a.m.

"I'd like you to do the preg checks on the beef herd down in Panguitch this year," he said, shuffling a pile of papers on his desk. "Probably good to get down there before the holidays."

I had never heard of Panguitch, or the fact that Utah State had a beef herd there. "Where's Panguitch?"

"South of here, down near the Arizona border. A couple hundred head run on that desert pasture. They round 'em up about this time each year, and our intern heads down to preg check 'em. Since they run with a bull, can't be sure when they were bred exactly."

A couple of hundred head of beef cows? I had zero experience with beef cattle while a student either at Penn or during my summers at Cornell. I pulled my bandana off, pushed the hair back from my face, and stared at him.

"We'll be sending an animal science student with you. She's grown up around beef cattle so she can teach you a thing or two" he said, chuckling. Of course, they had to find a girl. It wouldn't do to send a guy to help me.

My "preg check" skills were awful. For the last few months, whenever cows at the dairy needed preg checks, I followed

Dr. Nelson around trying my best to get the hang of it, but I still felt lost and increasingly discouraged.

"These cows and heifers will be at least two or three months pregnant," Dr. Nelson said, trying to reassure me. "Some of them will be much farther along. You'll feel a foot or a head," he laughed.

Didn't seem funny to me, and I sighed and stood up. "I guess it will be good experience."

"Don't sound so glum. You'll have fun."

The pep talk didn't help my confidence, but it was clear that I had to go. It would be an extreme form of on-the-job learning. The trip was scheduled for the following Wednesday. We'd drive south three hundred miles, preg check the herd Thursday, and drive back on Friday. That meant two overnights in Panguitch.

The day of the trip dawned cold and blustery—snow spit driven by a freezing wind. I packed my long underwear, warm wool hat and socks, heavy coveralls, and blue jeans. We would be working a long day outside. I sipped my scalding coffee but decided against bringing a thermos—what if the animal science student was a Mormon? She would roundly disapprove. Why Mormons disapproved of coffee I had no idea. In my house growing up, an old glass coffee percolator was always on the stove, ready to pour a cup for any friend who dropped by. Here, offering coffee was an insult.

The gray clouds were rushing over the snow-dusted Wasatch Mountains. I drove the truck up to the barn. Jeannie Riley jumped into the cab and tossed her backpack behind the seat. I smiled but she didn't. Jeannie must have been about twenty years old. Her long dark hair cascaded out of a stylish ski hat, and her tight blue jeans showed off her shapely legs. She wore a navy turtleneck covered by a green down vest, which highlighted her green eyes. Even though it was early morning, she had taken care to do her eye makeup, emphasizing her long lashes. Her cowgirl boots were authentically scuffed and worn. She turned and gave me a quizzical look. She had never seen a lady vet before. We stared at each other.

"You been down to the Panguitch herd before?" I asked, pulling out of the driveway.

"Once last year, with Dr. Nelson," she said.

"You grow up around here?"

"Yup. Grew up on a cattle ranch over in the Wind Rivers," she said. The Wind River Mountains were east of Logan, in Wyoming, wild and remote.

"My dad and granddad ranched there forever. Came West with Brigham Young from Ohio."

Over the course of the long drive south on Interstate 15, she chatted, and I drove. She had a steady boyfriend, a cowhand on her dad's farm, but they weren't engaged. Her Dad wanted her back on the ranch to be part of the family business. He was proud she was getting an animal science degree, but he expected prompt marriage and babies to follow once she graduated. She wasn't so sure, but since she had never been east of Kansas, she didn't have many ideas about what else she might do with her life.

Tossing her hair, she said, "Andy, that's my boyfriend, tried to give me a ring, but I just said, not until I graduate. Plus, I'm not sure he is the one, you know what I mean? I love him and all, but sometimes, I just don't know, he's so dull. My girlfriends all say I'm crazy, because he's such a looker, but you know, looks ain't everything. He's gonna be a deacon in the church someday for sure. Me, I still like to sneak a drink now and then—don't you tell!"

It was going to be a long drive.

❖

I listened to Jeannie's chatter as we headed south out of Salt Lake. The grandeur of Utah rolled out before us, wide open space, mountains in the distance. Driving past Provo, I could see the golden Angel Moroni with his trumpet perched on top of a Latter-day Saints temple tucked against the Wasatch Mountains in the eastern distance. We drove through high open desert, dotted with sage, Indian paintbrush, and a few sparse patches of dry, golden grass. West of Fishlake National Forest, there were a hundred miles between tiny towns with names from the Book of Mormon— Nephi, Manti. Towns too small for a temple, full of history of early settlements and the Pony Express, surrounded by masses of red rock, under a wide deep-blue sky. Bright sun, chilly wind, and the quiet of the truck rolled us along for long stretches without another car on the road.

With just one pit stop, we managed the 325-mile trip in just under five hours—the old vet truck was not built for speed. Panguitch felt empty when we pulled into the Blue Pine Motel. It was an old west town, with a wide main street lined with a drug store, the post office, gas station, and a store selling cowboy boots and hats. There were only two named streets in town—Main Street and Center Street. Like most Utah towns, the streets were numbered. The Church of Latter-day Saints was at 200 North 400 East, the most important address in town. Blue Pine was the kind of motel where each room had a door to the parking lot. We checked in at the cramped, dark office, scuffed linoleum on the floor, a framed picture of the Mormon Temple in Salt Lake on the wall. The motel guy, old and stooped, took a close look at these odd-looking girls checking into his motel.

"Where you ladies from?" he asked.

Jeannie said, "Logan. I'm in school up there. She's the vet come down to preg check the Utah State herd."

"The what?"

"The vet. We're going out to the ranch tomorrow." Jeannie raised her voice.

"Well, my heck! I ain't ever seen a lady vet. You a real vet?" he asked.

I affirmed I was real.

"Well, my heck," he repeated, smiling.

The sun was below the horizon and a sliver of moon rose in the clear cold sky. Behind the motel you could see off across the dry desert, where the shadows of mountains were barely visible. We were twenty miles from the main highway, and Panguitch was quiet in the way it's quiet in the desert. Dr. Nelson had told us to share, as his budget for the trip was tight. We hauled our backpacks into the room with two twin beds covered with thin blue flannel blankets pulled tight, peeling flowered wallpaper and one of those tiny ancient TVs with a rabbit-ear antenna.

Hands on the small of my back, I leaned forward and back, to shake off the stiffness of the long drive.

"I'm starving," Jeannie declared. She rummaged in her purse and pulled out a deep red lipstick which she applied, staring at herself in the mirror.

"Me too," I said.

"You should comb your hair," she suggested, frowning at me.

"Hopeless," I laughed. She cracked a smile.

The Rambler's Café was a block from the motel and featured chicken-fried steak and gravy, biscuits, meatloaf, and hot beef sandwiches on Wonder bread. They served Coke or coffee if you asked, but with a frown of disapproval. Pie for dessert, your choice of butterscotch or banana cream. The cow work would start early in the morning. It had been a long drive. Jeannie and I settled into the narrow beds. The cowboys at the ranch expected us at six a.m.

❖

The next morning there was hoarfrost on the truck windshield. The wind rattled through the flimsy walls of our room. We geared up, long underwear under our coveralls, wool socks, and wool hats. The ranch was thirty minutes out of town, and we pulled into a wide-open area with the cattle penned up and ready.

Five Utah cowboys, slim and muscled, were standing by a table, munching on powdered jelly donuts. They tried not to stare when Jeannie and I climbed out of the truck.

"Morning, ladies," one of them shouted. "You Doctor Rhodes?" he asked, turning to me. Good guess that the one with lots of lipstick and eye makeup was not the lady cow vet.

The breakfast was watery juice and supermarket donuts. Of course, no coffee. The guys were too busy sizing up Jeannie and her tight blue jeans to pay much attention to me. Apparently, they had been warned that a lady vet was going to be doing the preg checks, so they were more curious than surprised.

A couple of hundred beef cows were penned into a large corral, hooves churning the mud into a smelly soup.

"Let's get started," I said. The cowboys nodded and moved into their assigned places. We had a long day ahead of us. The first cow came barreling down the passageway. They caught her head in the metal clamp of the chute and pushed down the lever to squeeze her enough that she was unlikely to kick.

"Okay, she's all yours," one cowboy said. He wrote down her ear tag number and waited for me to declare her pregnancy status. Jeannie squirted lube on my long plastic sleeve. I squeezed through the fence, stepped in behind the cow and shoved my arm up her rectum, praying I could feel the uterus. She bellowed and strained, squeezing down on my groping arm. After what seemed like an hour but was only a few minutes, I thought I felt the top of the uterus with a bony thing inside. I yelled, "Pregnant!" and the cowboys let her go and pushed cow number two into the chute. One down, about two hundred to go.

If the cow's tail was manure soaked, Jeannie grabbed it so I wouldn't get slapped in the face. When my plastic sleeve tore after a couple of dozen cows, she handed me a new one. The cowboy kept records and looked increasingly annoyed. I groped and sweated.

"At this rate, we'll never get through the herd before dark," he said, watching me struggle with a fractious heifer. "Can't you speed it up?" The heifer let loose a tremendous pee sooner than I could dodge it. I felt the hot urine wet my leg and pool inside my rubber boot. At least it was warm. Her uterus felt small, so I yelled, "Not pregnant!" The heifer bolted out of the chute, and the cowboy muttered, "That one goes to McDonalds." Any cow that was not pregnant would go for slaughter. I took a sharp breath. Had I mistakenly killed the heifer with a misdiagnosis?

We slogged, some cows easy, some impossible. I knew I was making mistakes, but we had to keep going. There was no do-over here. At the lunch break, I went to sit in the truck alone, leaned my head on the steering wheel, and closed my eyes. Not halfway through and I was spent. Jeannie brought me a white bread ham and

American cheese sandwich and handed it in through the window without saying a word. I watched her chatting and flirting with the cowhands while I gulped it down.

We somehow made it through the entire herd, but barely before the sunset, when the temperature dropped to way below freezing. My feet were damp and cold from pee and sweat, my wool hat stained with manure where a stray tail had slapped me. I don't know what the cowboys thought, and I didn't care.

"Okay, ladies, have a safe drive home," the recordkeeper said. The others were gathering up their gear and heading to their trucks. The cows were in the large corral where they gulped down chunks of alfalfa hay torn from the bales the guys had thrown. My left arm was so sore I couldn't drive—Jeannie had to take over on the way back to the motel.

"You did good," she said, looking over at me slumped in the passenger seat.

"I was awful," I said. My eyes stung with tears.

"No, you did fine. Just slow," she laughed. I shrugged.

"A hot shower will fix you up," she said, pulling into the motel. "I'll run down to the diner and get takeout."

The next morning, on the long drive back to Logan, I thought long and hard about the preg checks. I knew some were guesses, but in some heifers I felt the pregnant uterus, some big with calves inside, some the size of basketballs. There was no way through this except practice, and more practice. At least I hadn't given up.

CHAPTER 20

THE CHRISTMAS OF 1978 WAS ice cold, with more than a foot of snow on the ground. Our small scraggly tree was decorated with a string of white lights I found at the Salvation Army and some cheap red balls that I bought at the last minute in the discount aisle of the grocery store. Dr. Nelson was out of town visiting cousins in Kansas. I had to stay close to the phone to cover emergencies. Vincent got up early and made a fire in the little woodstove while I dozed in the warm waterbed. Logan meowed for breakfast in the kitchen.

"Want coffee?" Vincent called.

"I'll get up," I said.

Vincent had plugged in the tree lights and put a wrapped present under the tree, next to the couple of presents that my mother had mailed to us. He handed me a mug and I stood on our rag rug by the woodstove warming my legs. Logan crawled under the tree and went to sleep among the presents. Vincent sighed.

"You okay?"

He nodded. I knew he missed his family at Christmas, the big Italian family gathering, his mother cooking homemade pizza, stuffed shells, roast chicken, the nieces and nephews quarreling over presents, the grandfathers sitting in armchairs drinking bourbon, chatting in Italian. If we had more money, he could have flown back to Rochester. We didn't. Neither of us felt like opening presents.

"Maybe next year we'll be in Rochester," he said. I thought about all the failed job interviews I had in New York State. I was busy doing my job at the university and hadn't allowed myself to worry about next year. And yet, we both wondered what might be next after my internship was over.

Finally, we opened the presents. I gave Vincent a new Swiss Army knife, and he gave me a green wool scarf and matching hat. After French toast and scrambled eggs, Vincent settled into the old couch and strummed his guitar. I called Josie and Dusty.

"I've been sewing ornaments," Josie said. "Little felt ornaments, with colorful embroidery." Josie was an expert embroiderer and created amazing abstract wall hangings and jazzy quilts.

"Kinda small project for you."

She sighed a deep sigh. "I don't have the oomph to tackle a big project. This way I can finish one beautiful, small thing, and it doesn't wear me out."

Most of the time I tried not to think about Josie's breast cancer. We told each other what we got for Christmas, and I thanked her for sending me the warm socks and down vest.

"Love you," she said, her voice catching. I hated that I couldn't hug her.

"Love you too." I hung up and went into the kitchen for more coffee. "I'll probably need to go visit soon," I said.

"Don't wait until she's too sick to enjoy a visit," Vincent said. Two weeks' paid vacation came with the job, but I didn't see how I could use it unless I talked Dr. Nelson into covering emergencies.

After breakfast, I lay down for a nap, praying that no one from the dairy would call. As I drifted off, cinnamon scent from the breakfast French toast lingering in the air, I heard Vincent talking to his brothers, laughing, happy.

"I know," Vincent said. "Next year." God, I thought. Next year. Back East. No job. The waterbed sloshed gently, and I fell fast asleep.

Later that afternoon, my sister called, worried. She had talked to Josie and Dusty too. "She sounds sad and weak," Anne said. "I couldn't get a word out of Dusty."

"I know," I said. "We should have both gone to California for Christmas." She and I were both thinking that it might be Josie's last.

"And Vincent is missing his music," I said. "He doesn't talk about it, but Utah just is not working for him."

"Linda, women follow men around for their jobs all the time," Anne said. "He can last another half a year."

"Yeah," I sighed. "I guess so."

Night fell early after a short day, the light faded into navy blue on the mountains, the snow glistened, the wind howled down Logan Canyon. I read Dickens's *A Christmas Carol*. Vincent worked a tricky tune out on his mandolin. Logan stretched full out as near to the woodstove as he could get without burning his fur. Sleepiness crept over me, even though I had a nap. I stretched and yawned. Vincent smiled, put his mandolin down and gave me a hug, and then a real kiss, the lingering kind. We ended Christmas early to bed, trying not to worry about what came next.

❖

In early February, Josie called to let me know at Dusty's regular physical exam, his doctor heard an alarming heart murmur. Once the cardiologists completed their tests, they recommended an aortic valve replacement surgery as soon as possible. The doctors were so alarmed that they scheduled open heart surgery for the following week. I thought of my father as solidly healthy, and this news was hard to process.

"You want me to fly out?"

"I think Dusty will need more support when he gets home from the hospital," Josie said.

"Are you sure? You don't want me there for the surgery?" I had two weeks paid vacation, and I wanted to spend it wisely.

"No, no," Dusty was on the phone extension in the kitchen. "He'll have plenty of care in the hospital and limited visiting hours."

"When I get home, it'll be a while until I can get around. I'll need some company," Dusty said. We agreed that after the surgery, I would fly out and spend two weeks with them. That would give me time to arrange with Dr. Nelson to take on the emergencies. I looked forward to some California warmth and sunshine.

The surgery was on a Monday. Josie called to let me know that everything went well. Dusty was pumped full of pain medication and getting good care. The next Wednesday, I sat in my quiet office and sorted through piles of journals and junk mail. Bitter cold had settled in the valley. That morning, I did my rounds at the dairy and sheep farms, but no one had anything for me to do. Soon it would be time for the lambs to be born, but now everything was quiet. The sound of the phone startled me. I picked it up, hoping it wasn't an emergency that would force me out into the cold again. Josie's voice made me sit up in my chair. My heartbeat quickened, thinking of Dusty in the hospital and all the possible bad things that could happen.

"Everything okay?"

"Dusty's fine," she said. I heard the tension in her voice.

"Thank God, I hate having him in the hospital when I'm not there."

"It's me that's the problem. I hurt my back. Rotten timing." Josie seldom complained about anything.

"What happened?"

"I don't know. I was getting a massage, and I felt something snap. It hurt like hell." I heard her strangle a sob. "Linda, it's really bad. I can't even bend over to feed Polo. I had to open the can and just dump the food on the floor. I don't think I can drive." I thought I heard her crying. "I have to get to the hospital, Dusty will be really worried if I don't show up."

I held the heavy receiver with the long black cord and paced. "I'll get a flight today," I said. "You need help."

"No, no, it can wait until you were planning to come out. Maybe I can get one of my friends to drive me."

"Josie, something is really wrong if you're in that much pain. We've got to get you to a doctor, and you should be in bed."

"Okay," she said, sobbing. "Okay."

After a rush of arranging for Dr. Nelson to take over my duties and buying a pricey last-minute plane ticket, Vincent drove me to the airport in Salt Lake City.

❖

Things in Altadena were worse than I expected. Josie, her thin skin pale, her shoulders bent, was in such pain that when I drove her to her doctor, every bump in the road caused her to cry out. The x-rays showed her breast cancer had come roaring back, metastasized to a femur, her skull and a vertebra. The massage therapist had fractured that fragile vertebra, causing the vicious pain.

The worried doctor told us he would set up appointments with a team of oncologists and get Josie on some strong pain meds. We were too stunned to cry. The next few days were a whirlwind. Josie was fitted with a splint to stabilize her back. Aggressive chemotherapy would start in a few days. She had to be in bed, or she risked another bone fracture.

The two weeks were a blur of shuttling among medical facilities. I visited Dusty in the hospital where he was recovering and then helped him to get settled back home. I drove Josie to the oncologists for more tests and her first session of chemotherapy. Insurance papers piled up, and each night I tried to make sense of the codes and claims. My sister Anne agreed to come out to California after my two weeks of what was supposed to be vacation were up.

The day before I had to go back to Utah, Dusty was propped up on the daybed in the living room, weak as a kitten, Polo with her paws tucked in on his lap. Josie dozed in the bedroom, recuperating from her chemo. The house was quiet, sun poured in the big windows that overlooked the garden.

"I hate to go," I said. Dusty was propped up with pillows, his pajamas hanging loose on his big frame.

"You have a job you worked hard to get—you can't walk away from it now," Dusty said. He put his big hand over mine.

"And Anne is coming tomorrow. She'll be a real help."

"I know."

Dusty was so pale. The long incision on the front of his chest where they cracked his ribs open was still red and raw looking. He sighed a deep sigh and coughed.

"Still hurts to breathe."

We sat in companionable silence. Polo, eyes closed, purring, was good company.

"It's Josie I'm worried about. She never complains, but the chemo is so hard on her." We both knew the return of her cancer was bad. Very bad.

"Maybe after you get back on your feet and Josie recovers from the chemo, I can get you both out to Utah. It's beautiful there," I said, petting Polo's soft gray fur. "You would love the Wasatch Mountains."

Dusty grew up in the Colorado Rockies, on the Western Slope where the Gunnison River ran wild and free through the Black Canyon.

He nodded. "I would like that."

Anne arrived the next day. After I oriented her on the pain medication schedule for both Josie and Dusty, the outstanding insurance stuff, the schedule for neighbors to bring dinners over, and the follow-up doctors' appointments, she drove me to the airport for my return flight to Utah.

I had done as much as I could.

CHAPTER 21

THE LONG LAMBING SHED WAS open to the bitter cold on one side. Two dozen ewes had been bred in the fall and with a five-month gestation were now ready to lamb. In early March, the temperature was still well below freezing at night. Powdery snow swirled where the drafts blew in between the wooden walls. Thick winter wool kept the sheep warm, but I shivered in my long underwear, jeans, flannel shirt, down vest, woolen cap, and old overcoat.

When I switched on the outside light, the dim bulb illuminated a hushed and expectant crowd of heavily pregnant ewes, sitting with their front legs tucked back under their chests, jaws moving slowly, rhythmically, back and forth, chewing their cud, hot breath misting from their round black nostrils. In the low light, I inspected each ewe, with their pink turgid udders pushed out under their back legs, their heavy wool dirty with a winter's worth of grime, greasy with yellow lanolin. Sheep secrete lanolin from glands in their skin to make their wool coats waterproof. Humans purify lanolin as an ingredient in commercial moisturizers, but I loved to wipe my dry, cracked winter hands over their greasy backs, a no-cost hand cream in the barn.

I walked quietly through the group, illuminating each ewe's rump with my flashlight. They looked up lazily, just as sleepy as I was. It was only one o'clock in the morning—I had another five hours on lamb watch. My rubber boots made a crackling sound walking over the thick straw bedding. Crystal stars shone in the still, inky sky. A mother ewe was in the far corner of the shed by herself, a sure sign of labor.

I knelt down. She looked up at me, turned her head back toward her flank, gave a grunt, threw herself full on her side, then struggled up to her knees, pushing. I went to her back end and looked under her tail—a bit of bloody mucus, but no sign of a little lamb foot. If a lamb presented front feet first, the mother usually needed no help in the delivery, unless there were twins. But if I saw a nose without feet, or worse, a hind foot, then I knew I had work to do.

The ewe gazed at me with her huge brown, inscrutable eyes, burped up her cud, and chewed. I took off my gloves and felt her udder. It was bright pink, huge and hard, with two teats sticking out, engorged with milk. Cupping both hands around her udder, the blood came back to my tingling fingers. Calm now, she didn't appear to be fully in labor. I would come back and check on her in a bit. I walked through the rest of the flock. No one else looked ready to give birth.

This was my first experience at lamb watch, a practice as old as agriculture, celebrated in the Bible: "And there were shepherds living out in the fields nearby, keeping watch over their flocks at night." The shepherd walks among the sheep, checking every hour for signs of ewes in distress, and helps deliver lambs that otherwise might die in birth. When the days shorten in the fall, the females (ewes) come into heat to attract their mates (rams). This is nature's way of assuring that lambs will be born in the spring, when the new grass can nourish their mother, so she can make the milk to feed them. And here in the barn, five months after they were bred, these girls were ready to give birth. We would have a few months of suckling lambs, weaning and then enjoying the summer before the days would again shorten and the cycle repeat.

I returned to the warmth of the barn office, where a box of seriously stale doughnuts hardened on the counter, next to the thermos of coffee I brought with me, a notebook for recordkeeping, and a narrow cot with a filthy pillow for the lamb watcher to lay down between checks. My boots were dirty with straw bits and sheep manure. I pried them off, left them by the door, pulled off my coat and wool hat, and flopped down on the cot. The alarm was set for two a.m., and it was already one-thirty. Pleasantly warm, smelling of sheep shit and straw, the little office was completely quiet except for the ticking of the wall clock.

❖

Over six months since I started, I worried about what came next in May when my internship was over. Yes, I was more experienced than a new grad, but my cow pregnancy diagnosis skills were still rudimentary. I had no real-world dairy vet experience, just the bit of practice I got at the university. Vincent still wanted to go back East and expected me to find a job there, but I didn't think my New York State large animal job prospects would be any better than they were ten months ago when I was a new graduate. Those old vets would be no closer to accepting a woman associate, even one with a year's experience. The internship was rushing by so fast that it was time to start a new job search, but I dreaded a repeat of the previous year's dozen failed interviews, so I put it off. Just thinking about it made me tired. Maybe Dr. Jacobs would take me back to his small animal practice in Pasadena if I got desperate. He had told me I was welcome back anytime. At least I would be making a salary to pay off my loans.

I nodded off. Too soon the alarm rang, time for the walk-through. My head hurt. Despite the warm office, I was chilled—the cement floor was always cold. I gulped a sip of coffee from my thermos, grabbed my flashlight, and went out to the shed. The ewe in the corner was straining, a pool of bloody, slippery, yellow-tinged fluid pooled behind her butt. I propped the flashlight under my chin to free my hands. When I raised her tail, there they were—two small front legs and a little nose, poking two inches out of her vulva. She strained, and the lamb's little face appeared, eyes squeezed shut, the tiny pink tongue lolling out the side of its mouth.

Excellent! Nice pink color! Correct position!

I don't know why I was so excited by a routine lambing, but giving birth never seems routine to me. The ewe let out a strangled roar—a sound that a sheep should never make—and pushed. The lamb flopped out on its side onto the straw, wet and slimy, little white ears plastered to its head with mucus. The ewe switched her tone to a mellifluous murmur, struggled to her feet and turned to give her baby a thorough licking. My role was to stand aside. If all went well, in another few minutes the lamb would be up and nursing, long tail wagging furiously. My interference at this point could result in the ewe rejecting the lamb, and then I would be bottle-feeding round the clock.

It was the darkest part of the night. The stars seemed to dim. I turned off my flashlight, sat on the crackly straw and listened to the ewe's rhythmic lamb licking, my breath misting in the cold. I leaned back against the fence, stuck my legs out in front of me, and sighed. This cozy shed and white, eager newborn lamb were so peaceful. There was no need for my professional services here. Everything normal, as it should be. I thought of my mother, and her mother before her, birth after birth, and my womb, waiting.

After the three, four, and five a.m. walk-arounds, I washed my boots in disinfectant, tidied up the cot and pillow, and wrote my notes in the log (one normal lambing, ewe #458, lamb nursing at three a.m.). Home to a shower and a couple of hours nap before I had to get to work sounded good. Lightheaded with lack of sleep, I settled into my truck, felt the heater kick on, and warmed my toes.

Almost a decade ago on the California commune, I learned how to flip a sheep so I could shear her, clipping the dense waxy wool off in clumps. The sheep went from fat and woolly to skinny and naked looking, with a couple of bloody nicks where I was careless with the clippers. But if a sheep had an odd lump, or was coughing, we had to call the vet. Now, I was the vet, a whole textbook of sheep facts stuffed in my head, diseases, anatomy, parasites. But most of it was just that—book knowledge. I needed more of what I was getting here in this grimy shed.

The veterinary intern didn't need to participate in lamb watch. Previous interns hadn't—they waited for the staff to call if there was a problem. Usually there were two or three calls per week for ewes in trouble during labor. I could have waited for the calls too, but I wanted to show the old guys at the sheep barn that I had grit, that I was willing to do the tough all-night work, in the cold.

I signed up for a couple of lamb watches a week, but any nights were more than the previous male interns. I had checked the sign-up calendar on the wall at the barn. I heard that the students thought it was crazy a vet would stay overnight in the lambing shed. Dr. Nelson told me it wasn't necessary.

"The guys will call you if there is a lambing they can't handle," he said. "They got a chuckle out of you spending the night on that grubby cot."

I didn't want them to know I had no lambing experience. I needed to see dozens of normal lambings in all their stages—the sounds, the smells, the timing—so I could know better when something was abnormal. The sheep barn guys knew so much more than I did, and I felt seriously foolish asking them how long I should let a ewe labor before declaring she needed help, how long I should let the lamb struggle to find the teat, how much bleeding during labor was normal, how much was alarming. That night, communing with mothers in labor, in the stillness and cold, I also knew I wanted to be there to experience the miracle of birth, a wonder in its own right, no matter the species, and a privilege to witness.

CHAPTER 22

WHEN SPRING CAME TO CACHE Valley and the mountains greened up after a few drenching rains, Doc Nelson walked into my office and said that his sister was sick out in North Dakota and that he'd be taking a week off to tend to some family business. By this time, he had the confidence to leave me on my own. We talked about follow-up treatment for a couple of cows at the dairy and discussed a prize ram at the Sheep and Goat Institute with a sinus infection that wasn't getting better. He turned to leave and said, casually, "Oh, and I gave them your emergency call number, just in case anything happens down at the bull stud barns while I'm away."

"When was the last time you had an emergency there?"

"Can't remember. The place is always quiet."

Good, I thought.

"They're used to taking care of most things that come up on their own. I'd be surprised if you hear from them, but you know, just in case."

❖

Late that Thursday afternoon, I was in my office when the phone rang.

"Hey Dr. Rhodes, it's Jeb here." I couldn't place the name.

"Jeb? Are you at the dairy?"

"No ma'am. I'm down at the bull barn. Can't find Doc Nelson."

Oh, right. That Jeb. "What's up?"

"You gotta find him, and he needs to come RIGHT NOW! We got

a bull down here that is bleeding mighty bad." I could hear the panic in his voice.

"Jeb, listen, Doc Nelson is out of town. What's happening down there?"

I heard him groan, "Okay, then, you come. Can't talk. Gotta get out there. Honk when you pull up, and I'll let you in." He hung up.

Bleeding really bad. Let's see. Sutures, largest gauge I have. Bandages. Cotton. Ropes. What else? Fluids. The drive was a blur, and I realized I hadn't checked for tranquilizer in the truck, but it must be there. I always kept a bottle. I screeched up to the office building honking the horn. Jeb came running from the back.

"Okay, come on."

"What happened?" I asked, jumping out of the truck and opening the back to grab my equipment.

"Bull got cut up really bad, bleeding like a stuck pig. Tried to attack a front loader!" He grabbed my gear, and we dashed around back.

I didn't hear the full story until later. One of the old guys who mucks out the stalls saw the whole thing happen. A new employee locked the bull into his stall and opened the back gate into the concrete pen outside. He drove the small yellow front loader into the pen to scrape the manure, just how he had been taught. The pens each have a door where the bottom and the top can be closed independently. Often, while the bull is restrained in the stall, the top half of the door is left open for fresh air.

This bull could see the little front loader coming into his territory—and he didn't like it. The problem was the new guy neglected to put the steel reinforcing bar across the lower door to the pen. Without the bar, the door shattered after only a couple of large head butts, and the bull was in the pen, challenging the little yellow front loader for dominance. He wasn't going to cede one inch of his territory to some little party toy of a machine. When the bull charged, the terrified worker jumped off and barely missed being crushed by the angry bull/front loader combination. He scrambled over the fence. The bull put his head under the blade of the front loader and shook his mammoth neck back and forth in a magnificent display of dominance. The front loader blade was sharp steel and at each shake, the blade bit into the skin and then the neck muscles of the crazed bull who ignored what must have been significant pain. Finally, the overwrought beast lost enough blood that he collapsed.

By the time I ran up, blood had spurted and pooled into a shallow lake on the concrete.

"Over here!" a cowboy yelled.

The bull's tremendous bulk heaved as he sucked in air. He lay on his side, eyes closed, his enormous chest moving up and down. One look and I realized no tranquilizers were needed—the bull was almost dead from blood loss. If I gave him fluids to get his blood pressure up, he would bleed more but maybe revive—and kill me. If I didn't, he might die soon. Fear and possibilities—too many possibilities—raged in my head. The whole crew quieted down, watching to see what would happen next.

Bleeding was the most critical thing to consider. I knew I had to stop it before anything else. Packing the huge wound would give me time to think. I climbed into the pen and walked around the great bull's head, wading through a puddle of clotting blood to look down into the gaping hole that had been carved by the front loader blade. The cut was about a yard long, curving over his massive neck, and at least ten inches deep, through layers of large muscles.

Multiple blood vessels spurted little red fountains. The entire wound was awash in blood. No possibility of neatly tying off the bleeders. At least it looked clean—a clean cut from a steel blade, no manure or embedded dirt. I didn't have enough cotton or a big enough needle. The supplies I needed were in the truck.

"Jeb, I'll be right back. You get some hot water."

I sprinted to the truck and pulled out rolls of cotton, needle holders, a package of heavy-duty catgut and the biggest curved suture needle I could find and dashed back.

"What do you want me to do?" Jeb asked.

"Does he need blood?" one of the technicians yelled.

Of course, he needs blood, I thought, but there is no goddamned cattle blood bank to call.

"You gonna give him a shot?"

"You need iodine?"

Everyone had a suggestion or opinion. I ignored them, knowing I had to handle this and make sure no one got hurt in the process. I ripped open several rolls of cotton and stuffed them into the wound. They disappeared. Two more, then two more. Finally, the blood stopped gushing.

"Jeb, lean on this cotton with your arms."

He nodded, climbed on the bull's back and sat there like a bull rider, leaning both his big forearms on the cotton rolls, starting to soak red. Maybe I could get some stitches in and then start IV fluids. The bull was not dead yet—I could see he was still taking shallow breaths. I threaded the large surgical needle with the catgut and cut off about a yard. I tried to act calm, but my hands shook. My mental picture of this bull waking up from the pain of me plunging the big needle into his neck muscle was terrifying, but there was no time for a local anesthetic. Jeb had been leaning on the cotton rolls for about five minutes, and the worst of the bleeding had slowed. I gingerly reached into one side of the wound and removed enough blood-soaked cotton to get a stitch deep into the interior muscle. I tried to remember the suture pattern that would take the most tension. The thick muscle pulled together as I tightened a big suture and tied a sturdy surgical knot, and then another and another—individual sutures for strength.

At least the first madness of the emergency was under control. My suture job wasn't pretty, but it stopped the bleeding. After fifteen minutes I finished suturing the deep muscle layer. At each bite of the needle, I pulled some of the blood-soaked cotton out of the wound. The technicians watched, standing outside the pen, peering through the steel fencing. The bull's breath was shallow and ragged, but he was still breathing.

The skin next, sutures not pulled too tight, but tight enough to close the wound. The leathery skin was much harder to sew, and

I discarded a couple of needles because they blunted from poking through that tough hide. The big rough catgut was the biggest suture material I had ever used—it felt like twine. I was about two inches away from finishing the skin suture across the wound when I heard the bull snort and stir. After so much blood loss, how could he wake up without fluids? He would be one sick bull unless I could get some into him before he completely woke up.

"Who can run to my truck and grab some fluids?" Jeb was still mounted on the bull, dabbing the remaining blood that was leaking from the wound.

"What do you need?" one of the guys asked, and I told him where to find the bags—I needed as many as he could carry. I threaded the needle with more catgut to finish the last few inches of stitches when the bull opened his eyes.

Jeb yelled, "He's waking up!" and deftly jumped off the bull's back and over the fence. I grabbed my needle holder and took a step back as the bull heaved himself to his feet. My initial sense of relief—*He's alive!*—was rapidly followed by *Oh shit*.

The groggy bull could barely stand. He looked around the familiar pen, turned his head and saw me. Even in his weak and wobbly state, his testosterone-crazed brain said, *Charge!* He swiveled toward me and lowered his head into attack posture. Each of my carefully laid sutures popped with a loud crack as he flexed his neck down, and I watched the incision gape open again.

"Run!" Jeb yelled, but I was already flat out.

I vaulted over the fence just as he crashed into the steel poles. The ground shook, and the bull went down in a heap. He had knocked himself out. I grabbed the fluid bags the tech had brought from the truck and jumped back into the pen. His wound oozed blood. At least my sutures had slowed the bleeding. I didn't know how much time I had before he woke up again, but I was determined to get some fluids into him. Jeb was right there with me, holding off the giant jugular vein while I plunged the needle in, hooked up an IV, and climbed up on the fence above the bull. Jeb and I sat up there, taking turns holding the fluids and changing the bags as they emptied. If the bull woke up suddenly, we'd both be on the right side of the fence.

The wound gaped open but the blood, thank God, was just a slow drip at the bottom corner. The suture job in the neck muscles was holding enough for the blood to clot, but my God, that wound was ugly. When the last fluid bag was empty, Jeb and I climbed down from the fence. With the big beast still unconscious, I took one more chance and went back in the pen to administer a mighty injection of penicillin—a full two bottles worth—and puff some yellow sulfa powder into the wound. Jeb and I looked at each other.

"You have a little blood on your face," he said, grinning. We both were soaked in blood, my glasses speckled red, hair clotting, coveralls smeared. I smiled.

"Let's see how long before this brute wakes up again," I said, expecting that he would wake up but knowing there was still a chance he wouldn't after so much trauma.

A long twenty minutes passed, and finally the bull heaved himself onto his chest, still too wobbly to stand, slowly moving his head, eyes blurry, from side to side. Maybe he knocked a bit of sense into himself and decided he had enough. He lay quietly, his breath ragged. By now, the late afternoon sun was low, the drama over. The poor new guy who had been on the front loader had gone to the emergency room for a tetanus shot. He'd been more than a little scraped up in the scramble.

I was a mess, sweaty and shaken from the ordeal. The worst of the blood clots and grime went down the drain at the deep sink inside the lab. Bull blood dried under my fingernails, and it would take a good soak in the tub to get rid of it. I didn't know where Jeb was, probably cleaning up in the men's room, I hadn't had a chance to thank him. I stripped off my coveralls, threw them on the floor of the truck cab, and climbed in to drive home.

Heading north up the valley, I didn't know if I had succeeded or failed. I went over the things I could have done differently and the things that could go wrong—infection, chronic draining wound, muscle damage, kidney failure. Sighing, I decided to call it a success for now. When I'd left, the patient was alive.

The story spread throughout Logan quickly. A bull attacking a front loader and then almost bleeding to death, combined with the lady cow vet handling the emergency, was big news. Doc Nelson returned the following week and heard most of the story at church.

"Heard you had quite a situation over at the bull stud place," was all he said.

"You chose the right time to be away."

Laughing, he patted my shoulder and said, "At least the patient lived, and no one got killed."

❖

A couple of months later, I drove south to see how my monster patient had fared. On tiptoe, peering into the bull's stall, I looked at the back of his neck. Amazingly, it had healed. A thick line of scar tissue ran behind his ears, and a deep V-shaped depression on his massive neck indicated where the cut from the front loader blade had been, but he moved easily around his stall, pawing and snorting.

I heard the door slam, and Jeb came down the hall.

"That's him, alright! Don't he look fine? Just as mean and feisty as ever!" Jeb reached out his thick hand and we shook. "You don't have to wait until Doc Nelson is out of town to visit again," Jeb said, winking.

"Please, no more emergencies."

"You got it, Doc."

I had earned that "Doc," and I was proud of it.

PART THREE

A Real Job

THE FIRST TIME I SAW Dr. Ron Hadley, it was a warm spring day near the end of my internship in 1979. He came down the hall by my office to deliver some milk samples to be tested for bacteria by the Utah State Diagnostic Laboratory. Ron's technician, Gail, trailed along behind him to fill out the paperwork. She wore white skin-tight shorts and a skimpy tank top, no bra, nipples prominent, her long blonde hair pulled into a tangled ponytail. Her saunter down the hall did not go unnoticed by the various men in the department, by whose open doors she passed. I heard her and Dr. Hadley laughing and looked out my office door.

Gail helped herself to a red hard candy from the bowl on the desk and sucked on it while she filled in the required information to submit the samples. Dr. Hadley spotted Dr. Marten in the hall and motioned him over for a chat. Dr. Marten must have said something funny, and I watched Dr. Hadley throw his head back with a loud guffaw, wink at Dr. Marten and give Gail's butt a pat.

"All done, honey?" he said. Dr. Marten looked down at the floor, and the secretary huffed and turned her back. Dr. Hadley reached for one of the red candies and popped it in his mouth.

"All set," she said. "They'll have the results on Monday."

"Great!" Dr. Hadley said. "Looks like you've gotten things going here, Dr. Marten. Used to take a couple of weeks for results. By then the damn cow could be dead!" He spit out another laugh. Saying "damn" in the halls of Utah State University was a grave offense, as was butt patting. A tall skinny man, Dr. Hadley had energy to burn and a quick, tense manner—he was taut as a stretched rubber band. He knew what he was doing now and had big plans for what he would be doing next.

Turning to leave, he saw me and waved. He turned to Dr. Marten. "She the notorious female intern?" he asked, loud enough for me to hear, tilting his head in my direction. Dr. Marten nodded.

"Hi!" Dr. Hadley shouted in my direction. "Come on over here and say hello." He waved me toward him with both hands.

"Clem, introduce me. Gail, you go ahead to the truck, I'll meet you there."

He looked me over. I was wearing a faded red short-sleeved t-shirt, blue jeans, old white sneakers, my hair cropped short. At five foot six inches, I had to look up to Ron's six feet. After nine months of large animal work, I was muscular and lean, proud of how strong I had become.

"How are you liking it here so far?" he grinned, and shook my hand with a muscular, ropy grip.

"I like it okay," I said. He was looking straight at me, and I could almost see him mentally flipping through the possibilities, trying to get a fix on what made me tick.

"Grow up on a farm?" he asked. "Dairy? 4-H?"

"No," I said. "I had cats growing up. Typical suburban childhood."

His bushy eyebrows went up, one higher than the other, and his thin lips curled into a smile. He thought he had me figured out, daughter of a dairyman or maybe a large animal veterinarian, smart and driven girl, with veterinary school as her goal growing up, finally fulfilling her dream in a man's world. Now he wasn't so sure.

Dr. Marten murmured something about having a phone call to make and left Dr. Hadley and me standing in the hall. Dr. Hadley bounced from one foot to the other, full of kinetic energy.

"You should come ride with me one of these days. I could show you some modern dairy practice, not like they teach it here at old Utah State."

"I'd like that."

"Gotta run. Gotta make a living. These academics, they get a paycheck no matter what they do. I gotta earn it." He trotted down the hall. I turned to go to my office when Dr. Marten came out into the hall.

"I wouldn't trust that guy, if I were you," he said. "Married man, always in here with one or the other of his girls, dressed like that." The secretary smirked.

I felt oddly attracted to Dr. Ron Hadley—his energy, his irreverence, his in-your-face attitude toward the Mormon faculty. *Cool guy*, I thought. *Very cool.*

❖

I can't remember when he offered me a job, but it must have been some time that spring when my internship was coming to an end.

"Dr. Hadley wants me to join his practice," I said. Vincent and I sat on the front stoop, in the late spring sunshine. He was picking out a tune on his mandolin. He put it down and sighed.

"You want to say yes, right?" He stared at the ground. I scooted closer and put my arm around his shoulder.

"What else can I say?" I asked. "There's not a chance I can find a cow job back East, you know that."

"You won't even try?" he said. Our eyes met and he stared at me. We both knew how badly he had hoped to return to Freeville, his brothers, their music, his family.

"How can I try? We don't have the money for me to fly back for job interviews in New York." I stood up and paced. "None of those practices will be any more welcoming now than they were a year ago."

"Why not?" Vincent asked. "You have so much more experience now."

"Not in the real world, only as an intern," I said. Logan rubbed my leg. I leaned down to pet him. Vincent sighed, picked up his mandolin and plunked out a minor chord.

I stared east up Logan Canyon. The icy water in the irrigation ditch was rushing down from the snowmelt in the mountains, and a fresh spring breeze blew white wispy clouds through the clear blue sky. The West felt like home to me—the Wasatch Mountains bookmarking the valley I now knew so well, the broad expanse of Cache Valley, green with alfalfa, dotted with dairies. Could I trade this for going back to Freeville, with no savings and no job lined up? Knocking on those unwelcome doors?

"I can't turn down my first real large animal job offer for the off chance that something will turn up if we move back East," I stated. "I just can't."

My stubbornness hurt us both. We were precariously close to losing a relationship I had tried hard to keep intact over the last decade. Wives accommodated their husband's relocation, following the husband wherever his job took him. Why was it wrong of me to reverse that old role and ask Vincent to follow me? And yet, if he wasn't happy, why should he stay? I knew I was stretching our relationship thin. How much tension could it take? So many questions. This job in Logan, taking care of cows, doing what I trained to do, was finally possible, and I couldn't turn my back on it.

❖

The Utah State campus bustled with students taking final exams, the weather warm for May. The snow on the Wasatch Mountains had melted until there were only small white caps on the peaks. My internship was almost over, and I was eager to start my new job with Dr. Hadley, where I would be out in the country with the local farmers. I had good experiences at Utah State—my first C-section, my first solo left displaced abomasal surgery that had turned into a theater-in-the-round for the local cowboys. My late nights in the lambing barns helped me feel more comfortable with problem ewe pregnancies, my preg check and cow palpation skills had improved. A year of internship had increased my confidence, but I still had a lot to learn.

Cows sixty days pregnant or later I usually got right, but earlier pregnancies eluded me. Ovaries were hard to feel too. I would get plenty of practice with Dr. Hadley, and that was all that was needed

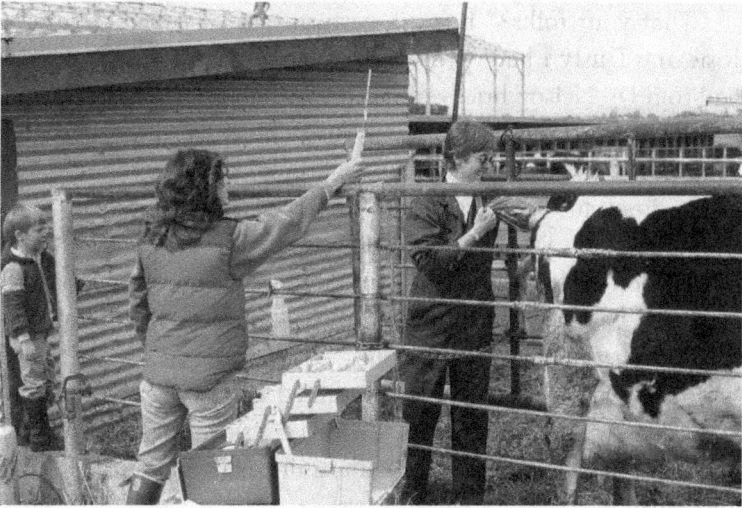

Rectal exams were often done outdoors. It helped to have a vet tech
assist to hand over a uterine catheter, with antibiotics. The fishing
tackle box held supplies. The dairyman's young son observed.

to become as skilled as I had to be, I told myself, trying to believe
it. Besides, I had long arms and long skinny fingers that made rectal
palpation easier for me than for the big male vets with thick arms
and stubby fingers. The lady cow vet advantage.

The campus emptied out as students finished their finals. A
warm breeze blew down the canyon. I walked over to the student
center for lunch, passing the building where Dean Anderson had
his office. If it had been up to him, I never would have been offered
the internship. I bet Dr. Nelson had to twist his arm. Maybe by
now he heard some gossip about the lady cow vet and how she did
a pretty good job, after all.

The last week of my internship, Dr. Nelson poked his head
into my office. "Looks like you are packing up." I boxed up my
vet journals and brought them home, and most of my textbooks
too. Now I was sorting through various papers and detritus left
in my desk.

"That your folks?" he said, gesturing to a framed picture of Josie and Dusty I had on my desk. "How's your mom doing?" I had told Dr. Nelson briefly about Josie's illness.

"She finished the chemo. It was rough but seemed to work. Her tumor isn't progressing as far as we know."

He shook his head, looking down. "My aunt went through it. Rough stuff."

"Listen," he said, looking up and smiling. "I've been wanting to talk with you, get your impression of the year here. Kind of sum things up before you leave. If you're not busy, we could talk now."

"Sure, that's fine." We seldom talked about anything but the latest illness at the dairy or a follow-up on a sick ram, or something related in one way or another to the animals in our care. This felt awkward.

"Good. Excellent," he said brightly. He sat down and swiveled his chair to face me. His blond hair, thinning at the temples, was neat with comb marks, his pressed white shirt looked freshly laundered. I wondered if his wife did his ironing, or one of his daughters. He sat up straight and cleared his throat. "First of all, I wanted to tell you that I've been pleased with your performance as an intern in this program." I sat back in my chair and looked down at my hands, feeling nervous. A performance review, then.

"You actually have been the best intern we have had in this program," he said, grinning at me. There was a beat of silence.

"Well," I said. "That is nice of you to say."

"No, really. You came with excellent skills, you paid attention to the things you needed to work on, you asked great questions, and I've never seen a harder worker."

Perhaps I should have just enjoyed the praise, but I couldn't help but comment.

"Maybe next time a woman applies for the internship, you'll be more open to considering her application, then." I was thinking about how they had thrown my application in the garbage the first time around and only accepted me out of absolute desperation. I smiled sweetly at him, to help the medicine go down.

He laughed quietly, shaking his head, the laugh relaxing into a smile.

Looking straight at me he said, "Oh, no, we won't take a chance on hiring a woman again."

I laughed, sure he was kidding. Then I looked at him, and he sat smiling at me, as if we were both enjoying the same joke.

"You are an exceptional talent, Linda, and we all enjoyed working with you." He nodded his head vigorously. "But I have talked to the other faculty and staff, and we don't think it likely that we would be so lucky a second time. No—we'll stick to the tried and true for the future."

My face reddened and I sucked in a deep breath. Dr. Nelson looked relaxed like he felt good about my end-of-internship evaluation. Clearly, he thought I would be happy with his praise. I realized my mouth was hanging open. Just then, Dr. Marten poked his head in the office.

"Lamar, we have to go over to the extension office for our three o'clock meeting. I've been looking for you."

"Oh golly!" Dr. Nelson said, jumping up. "Linda, so sorry, I plumb forgot I promised to go to Clem's meeting." Together, they walked briskly down the hall.

❖

I stared at the door and sank back in my chair. So that was it. If I made a mess of the internship, wilted under the pressure, cried when a cow kicked me, gave up and begged for help when I had trouble lifting a cow's foot for a trim, then for sure women shouldn't be trying to do large animal practice. But strangely, when I did none of those things but excelled far beyond anyone's expectations, well then, I was the exception that proved the rule. No other woman could do as well as I did, and why take the chance of hiring another one?

CHAPTER 24

DR. HADLEY HAD A BUSY practice with dairy farms in the north-east corner of Utah, up Cache Valley into Gem Valley, Idaho, and as far north as Lava Springs. Wildly busy and overextended, he needed another veterinarian. Thinking back, I expect that no other Utah vet was willing to work for him. He was quirky and, most damning, not a Mormon—maybe even an atheist. Although married, he had no kids, and worse, his wife, Kay, worked—she was a mathematician at Thiokol, the missile manufacturer in Brigham City. The dairymen were willing to hire him to take care of their cows for two simple reasons: he got results, and there were no other veterinarians within a hundred miles. Dairies that followed Dr. Hadley's herd health program had healthier cows, and healthier cows gave more milk and made dairies profitable. They could put up with his unconventional, irreverent self as long as he took good care of their cows.

My intern salary was twelve thousand dollars a year. Dr. Hadley offered me fourteen, which seemed generous. I was paying back my student loans at the rate of four hundred dollars per month, so there wouldn't be a lot of wiggle room in my budget, but a couple more thousand dollars a year would help. We agreed that he would buy me a truck and supply my equipment. He even bought me a washer and dryer, which seemed odd as a work benefit, but after a few weeks on the job, I understood—the pair were in constant use, washing and drying loads of coveralls, towels, and rags.

Dr. Hadley had a program: each dairy paid him a monthly fee on a per-cow basis. For that fee, he came a few times a month, performed routine preventive care, and attended to any cows that had health problems, such as lameness, mastitis, coughs, abscesses, or reproductive issues. Emergency work was included too, which meant that if he came out at night for a calving or had to show up in a snowstorm for a cow down with milk fever, the farmers didn't pay extra. Dr. Hadley was a better veterinarian than he was a businessman. This kind of preventive care program, called herd health, was rare at the time. Dr. Hadley was the first to use it in this part of the country.

"I've worked it out," he said. "Took me years to come up with it. If you work for me, you have to follow my plan." He was bustling around, loading up supplies in his truck. "My clients are all over Cache Valley, and my best are the Mickelsons, up in Grace, Idaho. A father and his three sons. Top-notch dairies," he bragged.

I nodded. Who was I to question? There was so much to master that it seemed wise to follow the lead of someone much more experienced. "Sure, of course," I said.

He winked and said, "Thatta girl," and I felt the frisson of excitement from his approval.

❖

I signed another year's lease on our little stone house. Vincent and I agreed that he would stay with me, at least for now. His new band was getting a few gigs, and summer was lovely in Cache Valley. Neither of us wanted to have the harder conversation about laying down roots in Logan.

"We'll just see how it goes," I said, taking the pile of coveralls out of the dryer. "With a bit of extra money, at least we can afford plane tickets back East."

"If you ever get any vacation," he said.

We had achieved a fragile balance, with me in a job I had dreamed of and Vincent making do in Utah with the musician friends he had found. The alternative? He could leave and go back to Freeville, settle in with his brothers and their music, and give up on me. He knew I wouldn't go with him and abandon my dream. We didn't

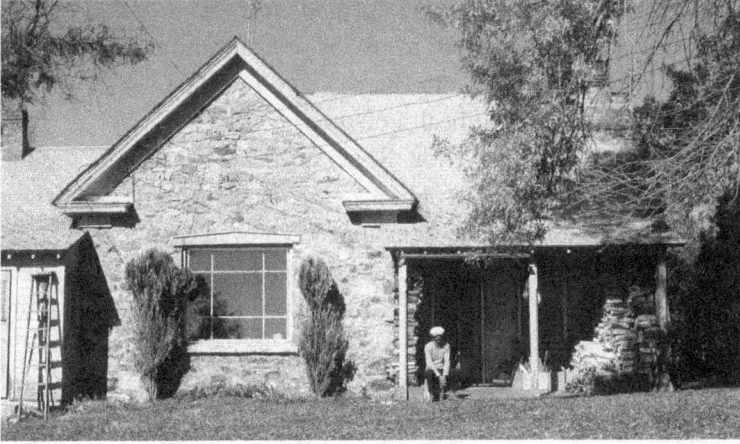

Vincent on the front porch of the stone house.

discuss it—Vincent was not much of a talker. Some days I felt defiant. Of course, I had a right to do the work I wanted. Vincent could adapt. We could find a balance. Other days, I felt guilty and selfish. No musicians in Logan were equal to his brothers, their tight family ties. His grandfather and father were both musicians, the three brothers growing up together, learning chords, singing harmony.

Perhaps this was when Vincent first considered leaving me, yet he had the same inertia I did. *A body at rest will remain at rest unless it is acted upon by force.* What that force might be, I had no idea.

❖

Dr. Hadley employed two technicians; Gail, who had worked in the practice full-time for several years, and Lee, an animal science student who wanted to be a veterinarian and rode with Ron part-time, fitting the schedule around her classes. Lee had blonde hair and blue eyes, like Gail, but that is where the similarity stopped. She was short and stocky, compact, her hair tied in a long, tight braid. Metal-frame glasses perched on her nose. While Gail seemed to work in languid slow motion, Lee was a whirlwind. That girl could get things done. Dr. Hadley had given them both a couple weeks off while he oriented me to his practice and introduced me to his clients. He saved some money, and I did the vet tech work while I learned his herd health methods.

For those few weeks I was Ron's sidekick. He showed me the ropes, quite literally. He taught me his trick knots to tie up a cow's head or a foot for a lameness exam. We enjoyed each other's company. I loosened up. He stood too close when we were leaning over a surgery together, hands gloved and bloody. He didn't slap my butt, but I thought he wanted to.

After long dirty days, driving home exhausted with muscles tired from solid work, we relaxed in the truck, drank Cokes and gossiped about the farmers, who, we were sure, gossiped about us. I was married to Vincent, Ron was married to Kay, but we saw less of our spouses than we did of each other. This was our honeymoon period. We both knew that in a few weeks, when the new Ramcharger truck he'd ordered for me arrived, we would hardly see each other. I would be working on one set of dairies while he went to another. That was the whole point—to be able to cover more territory and expand the practice.

And teach me he did. He took my textbook knowledge and converted it into skill, showing me high-quality shortcuts, simple practical ways of doing common things. I started moving more fluidly around the cows, with confidence. He noticed. I was proud.

"Let me show you a trick about an epidural," Ron said. We were delivering a breech calf, but the cow was straining so hard neither of us could get a grip on the second hind leg, folded back and difficult to reach. I drew up the lidocaine into a syringe. Although I knew how to do an epidural—I'd done one on the first C-section I did at the Utah State dairy—I wanted to see Ron's method.

"You move the tail up and down like this. Feel for this space right here."

His method was better. Clever, clean, no fumbling. Details of where he stashed equipment in his truck were carefully worked out. He thought ahead about what he might need and when, then placed the items where it made the most sense. I pictured him lying awake at night, staring at the ceiling, figuring out if the tetracycline bottles were better on the left or right side of the truck. My brand-new Dodge Ramcharger four-wheel drive truck with a custom cab was delivered, white, clean and full of power.

"What do you think, Doc? Big enough for you?" he crowed.

"It's great! I love it!" And I did. I'd never had a brand-new vehicle. It was a stick shift, room in the front for two passengers, a cooler for vaccines between the seats. The back was outfitted with milk crates holding surgical packs, drugs, ropes, fluids, catheters, coveralls—everything I needed.

The next day, I met Ron at six a.m. at the local diner for breakfast, ready to drive my new truck out to my first solo farm visits. Ron gave me a map on which he had circled my assigned dairy farms. Our table was littered with the remains of breakfast, half-eaten buckwheat pancakes, plates of scrambled eggs scraped clean, toast. I nursed my coffee, holding the mug in both hands, inhaling the steam.

"You start with the Otises' place and then go north through Smithfield. I'll go south through Nibley and Hyrum, it's on my way home." Ron lived in a town called Paradise, Utah, about twelve miles south of Logan.

"And what if I need to get in touch with you?" I asked. I'd gotten used to talking to Ron about every case and every cow, discussing diagnosis, methods, cases, approaches.

"Call my home number and leave a message with the answering service. I check my messages after each stop." An office secretary was a luxury that couldn't be justified. "We can call each other when we get home and make plans for tomorrow."

I speared the last home-fried potato on my plate. "Okay," I said, taking a deep breath.

"You ready?" Ron said, looking intently at me.

"Sure," I said.

❖

We were poor, I suppose, but I didn't feel poor now that I had a regular paycheck. We had enough money for the basics—food, rent, electricity, gas for the old Peugeot. Our sparse furniture was from the Salvation Army, the dishes hand-me-downs. Books we borrowed from the library, we seldom ate out, and there was no time or money for a vacation.

Vincent earned money here and there from his band gigs and part-time jobs he found. He helped a local contractor build shelving and workbenches for a small Logan company and installed gym flooring in a new phys-ed center at the university.

Given my insistence on financial equality in a relationship, we split expenses. We kept our own bank accounts. Mine was growing slowly, although there wasn't much surplus for savings given the crushing student loan payments I made every month.

While I was employed by Utah State, Vincent was covered under my health insurance. When I went to work for Ron, my compensation included my health insurance, but not Vincent's.

"The cost is about eighty dollars a month."

"What cost?" he asked. I had been talking about how Vincent would have to find somewhere to buy health insurance, and how much deductible was reasonable, and which plans included what. He had tuned out.

"For your health insurance. I can get it through the American Veterinary Medical Association."

"I don't want it. I'm not getting sick." True, he was a healthy thirty years old. I couldn't remember when he was last ill.

"But what if you fall skiing and break your leg?" I swiveled around from my desk and looked at him. "If you don't have insurance, it will cost more money than you can afford." I didn't snoop in his checking account, but I was sure he had almost no savings.

"I'd splint it up myself," he said. "You're a doctor, you could help." I stared at him. He shrugged. "We don't need any fancy hospital. Think about what the Native Americans did. They didn't have health insurance."

"That's just irresponsible," I snapped. I felt my face getting hot, and my hands clenching. This sounded like the beginning of a digging-in-heels kind of argument.

"Look, if you don't have health insurance, and someday you need medical care, you know what will happen?" I paced around the living room, waving my arms for emphasis. "I will pay the bills, and if I can't afford it, your parents will pay because you don't have any savings."

"I wouldn't ask you to pay."

"Of course you wouldn't. But the people who love you would not want you to go without medical care."

"Linda, don't get so worked up. I'm healthy. I don't need it." He put his hands on my shoulders. "You need it, because you have a dangerous job. I understand that. I don't want to waste money on insurance I don't need."

The argument went around in circles. I told him how expensive Josie's chemotherapy had been, how common unexpected medical bills are. He just stared at me. Finally, I gave up.

"Okay, I'll pay for your goddamned health insurance." I sat down and took out the AVMA form to apply.

"But you have to promise me if ever you need the insurance, even if it's for an ingrown toenail, you will pay me back in full for the monthly bills."

He laughed. "I promise." He wrapped his arms around my shoulders and looked at the form.

"Send it in so we don't have to fight about it anymore." He kissed me on the top of my head. "I'll be fine. I'm not gonna break a leg."

As I slipped the check and the completed form into an envelope, I muttered under my breath "Be healthy, Vincent."

CHAPTER 25

RON WAS EAGER TO TAKE some time off. After my first couple of weeks, he and Kay loaded up their two mules in a horse trailer and left for a two-week mule-packing trip in the Wind River Mountains in Wyoming, leaving me on my own.

Ron's dairymen were not ready for a new vet, particularly a girl. Gail disappeared as soon as Ron left, and Lee had classes, so my vet tech help was spotty. When I pulled up to Greg Mauchley's Idaho dairy, he was hosing down the manure in the holding pen. A stocky young guy, early thirties, already with five kids, he moved at a deliberate pace, not rushed but always busy. Blue eyes under a baseball cap, pulled low over his dirty blond hair, hands thick from cow chores, he walked over to the driver's side of the truck and peered in the window.

"Where's Doc?"

"He took off for a couple of weeks of camping."

"Took those mules with him? And the dogs, I bet," he said, shaking his head. Ron had three Australian Shepherds he doted on. "Where's Gail? You all by yourself?"

"Guess so," I said. I climbed out of the truck and went around to the back. I pulled on my dark green coveralls and high rubber boots.

"We might as well get started," I said, reaching for my equipment box and the stainless steel pail I used for hot water. Greg leaned down to pick up the box at the same time. Our heads almost touched.

He followed me into the barn. "Got the ladies in the holding pen. You want to get started?" Greg said.

And just like that, I transitioned to his veterinarian. We managed to get through the list—a cow with a cyst on her ovary got an injection, I diagnosed a sixty-day pregnancy. One cow had a discharge from her vagina that smelled rotten—she had a uterine infection and I gave her an injection of a new drug that had just been released.

"What's that stuff?" Greg asked, looking at the bottle.

"New drug that helps her clear out her uterus," I said. Now I smelled almost as rotten as the cow from her discharge dripping on my coveralls. "Causes the uterus to contract and push out the infection."

"Haven't seen Doc Hadley use this," he said, frowning. He shrugged, "If it helps Daisy to get back in calf, I'm all for it. She's one of my best milkers." I loved that Greg named all his cows.

"I think that does it," I said, pulling off my manure-covered rectal sleeve. I turned it inside out and dropped it in the trash bin. We had been working steadily for about an hour and a half. My arm was tired.

"Greg, can I ask you something?" I scrubbed my boots with my boot brush, getting the worst of the manure off. "Why is it that Mormons don't drink coffee?" I was hoping Greg wouldn't be put off by my asking. I knew that the Church of Latter-day Saints, or the LDS as the dairymen called it, didn't approve of coffee or Coke.

"You know who Joseph Smith is, right?"

"Of course I do," I said.

"We abide by the Word of Wisdom," he said. "Joseph Smith received the Word of Wisdom as a revelation from God in 1833, when he was preaching in Ohio."

"So this Word told the prophet that God didn't want people to drink coffee?"

"Not exactly," Greg said. "It prohibits wine, strong drinks, tobacco, and hot drinks."

"That covers a lot of territory."

"There's a lot of other stuff about what to eat to keep healthy,"

Greg said. "I can get you a copy of the Doctrine and Covenants. It's all explained in there."

"Thanks, Greg. Think I'll pass for now." All my dairymen clients had offered me copies of the Book of Mormon. I had accepted the first one and since had learned to say no as gracefully as I could.

"One more thing before you go," Greg said. "I have a girl out back in the hospital pen, off feed for a couple of days, not looking right." I didn't know it then, but Greg was a master dairyman and knew his cows better than he knew his kids. If he said something was "not looking right," you could bet that cow needed help.

I grabbed a stethoscope and thermometer from my bag and followed him. The warm barn was quiet, flies buzzed around the open door, a black-and-white cat darted out. The sick cow lumbered to her feet when we came in. She didn't look too bad to me. I started a physical exam.

"When did she calve?"

"About two months ago. Haven't bred her back yet," Greg said. He took his baseball cap off and rubbed his big hand through his hair. "Last couple of days she hardly ate anything."

My stethoscope on her lungs, I nodded. Heart and lungs sounded fine.

Behind her was a pool of watery diarrhea.

"You give her anything?"

"Nope, thought since Doc was coming, I'd wait for him to treat her."

I put my stethoscope over the cow's upper left side, back near her hip bone, just over her rumen, listening for that deep rumbling, gurgling, liquid sloshing that indicated normal rumination—nothing. Quiet as a church on Tuesday.

Greg stood back, watching. It was the first time he had ever seen a lady vet do a physical exam on a cow. I moved the stethoscope a bit down and forward on her left side, leaned over so I could listen, and with my thumb and forefinger, flicked her side as hard as I could. And there it was, that "ping" sound, so satisfying, so diagnostic. I flicked my finger again—just to make sure. I thought back to Craig, the dairy manager at USU who insisted Utah cows didn't get this condition. Even Doc Nelson had been surprised when I did the surgery and they saw it with their own eyes.

I straightened up. "She's got a twisted stomach."

Surprised, Greg frowned. "You sure?"

"Absolutely."

"So, she'll need a surgery?" he asked, walking over and patting her on the rump. "This old gal is one of my best milkers. I'm milking three of her daughters, all hundred pounders a day." He shifted his weight from one foot to the other a couple of times, took off his cap again, and dusted it on his dirty coveralls.

"Can it wait?" he asked.

"Can what wait?"

"The surgery. Can it wait until Doc's back?"

I looked at the cow. She didn't look too bad, but she was going to get worse, no telling how fast. "Shouldn't wait too long," I said, trying to sound sure of myself. "I can do the surgery, I've done a few on my own." But there it was. Either I did the surgery, or the cow would get sicker while we waited for Ron to get back.

Greg stared at me. Hard decision. One of his best cows. The lady cow vet. Doc gone. No other vet within a hundred miles. The flies buzzed. The cat trotted across the barn. I waited.

"Why don't you give her one of those pink pills, and we'll see how she gets on?" he said.

❖

Bone tired and constantly anxious, I dragged myself along, more irritated each day Ron was gone. Cache Valley was beautiful in June, the alfalfa greening up, the last of the snow gleaming on the mountains, but with no time off, I couldn't enjoy the weather. I was doing the work of two veterinarians. Some dairymen canceled their regular monthly appointments, but for emergencies, I was the only game in town. Those two weeks were cursed with an unusual number of middle-of-the-night difficult calvings and milk fevers. I grabbed meals when I could, drank coffee by the gallon, washed

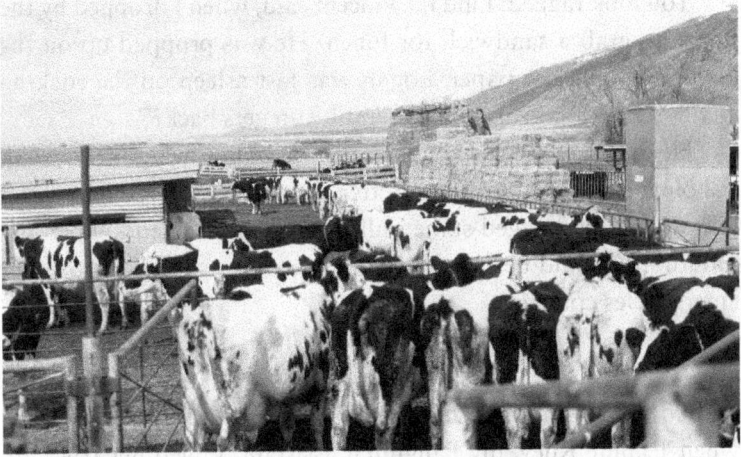

Holstein cows on a typical Utah/Idaho dairy. The hay is alfalfa
for feed. Idaho grows some of the best alfalfa in the country.

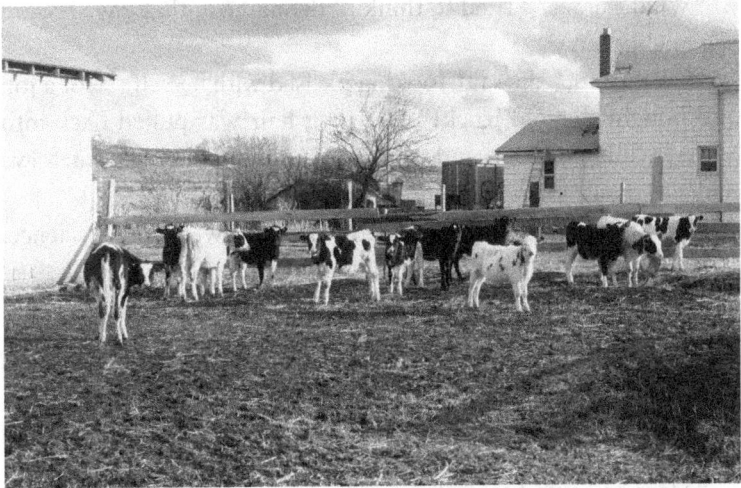

Young Holstein replacement heifers.

piles of manure-covered coveralls, drove at night and at dawn,
covering a practice area more than a hundred miles in diameter.
When I was home, I was either eating or sleeping. Vincent took
care of the cooking.

"You look ragged, Linda," Vincent said, when I dropped by the house to grab a sandwich for lunch. He was propped up on the couch, reading the paper. Logan was fast asleep on the rocking chair. "Can't some of this wait until Ron gets back?"

"He expects me to keep up the practice while he's gone," I said, gobbling a big bite of peanut butter and bread. "Don't want to let him down." I chugged some milk from the bottle and wiped my mouth. "I should be home by seven tonight as long as no other emergencies come up."

❖

Late in the afternoon, bone tired, I was filling the truck with gas when Jeannie Riley, my Panguitch assistant, pulled her truck up behind mine and waved. I hadn't seen her since last winter.

"Hey, Doc," she said. I walked up and put my elbows on her open window.

"What's new?" I tried to think of the name of that guy she said she might marry.

"Graduated," she said, looking pleased with herself. "Got a job and bought this old truck!" Her long hair was pulled back into a serviceable ponytail, and I noticed she didn't have as much eye makeup on as when we went to Panguitch together.

"Good for you," I remembered her major was animal science. "You working for your dad?"

"Not on your life. I figured if you could do a man's job, so could I." She winked at me. "I got a real job, down at the sheep farm at Utah State." I knew that barn. I had slept in the lambing shed. "They told me first time they ever hired a girl there."

"And what happened to what's his name?"

"Married some high school girl who's already pregnant," she giggled.

❖

By the end of the two weeks, I was proud of myself. I had managed the busy practice on my own, emergencies and all. The map Ron gave me, with his client's farms marked in red, was torn and dirty from all the times I had pulled over to the side of the road to consult it. Almost everything had gone well, except Greg Mauchley not wanting me to operate on his cow's twisted stomach. No patients had died. Our clients were talking to one another—that lady cow vet had done forty rectals at the Lewistons, had stitched up a torn teat at the Jenson farm, had delivered backward twins at Terry Chatterton's place, had given that newborn calf that was almost dead some kind of new medicine, and you know, that calf was up running around the next day!

I don't know what exactly I expected on Ron's return. A bonus, maybe a few hundred dollars, a couple of days off, plus a healthy amount of praise and gratitude. He could rely on me. I labored so he could have a rejuvenating vacation with his mules and his wife. Ron could see how busy I'd been, as all the billing sheets were filled out and stacked up on his desk. It was after dark on Sunday when he gave me a call.

"I'll head up to Grace tomorrow, and you'll be in the valley, right?" Meaning we will return to our normal schedule, including me working my normal six-day week and being on call Monday, Wednesday, Friday and Sunday.

"Back to the regular schedule?"

"Great trip. Did you fill my truck up with gas?" That was a job of one of the vet techs, not me.

"Nope," I said. "I don't believe anyone touched your truck while you were gone."

"Damn. I'll have to get up extra early then. Okay, talk to you later tomorrow."

"One thing, Ron. Greg Mauchley has an LDA cow that needs surgery. He's been waiting for you to do it."

"Okay, I'll add it to my schedule for this afternoon. Didn't count on that much work my first day back." I hoped Greg's cow had survived the wait.

And that was that. I plopped down on the old red couch. Vincent looked at me and raised an eyebrow—he'd been working all afternoon on plans for a custom plywood cabinet with drawers and shelves to make my gear fit better into the Ramcharger. Logan was fast asleep on the couch pillow. Shoulders hunched, jaw clenched, fists balled, I went out the front door. The evening was balmy, the breeze fresh with sage and cedar. The slim silver arc of moon barely visible against the black bulk of the Wasatch Mountains, sky a cerulean blue shading to indigo. I walked down the driveway, gravel crunching beneath my sneakers, up the path toward the irrigation ditch where I could hear the dark water rushing by, carrying snowmelt from the mountains.

I thought about what I needed. A word of thanks. A simple "good job." I was worn out, the last bit of my energy seeping away. I walked uphill toward the mountains in the total darkness. I climbed high enough that I could see the lights of our living room below, with the faint glow of the town of Logan farther down the valley. I sat in the dirt and sobbed.

CHAPTER 26

THE WARM SUMMER RAIN SPIT against the windshield, wind whistled up through Logan Canyon. The leaves of the oak trees gleamed in the damp. Low pearl-gray clouds settled in the valley. In the center of town, the white steeples of the Church of Latter-day Saints glowed against the darkened sky. I pulled into the driveway and shut off the truck. Lee and I sat for a minute in companionable silence, listening to the rain falling on the roof. She sighed.

"I'll stock up the truck," she said.

The house was quiet. After being up since four a.m., and with rain pattering against the windows, I considered a late-afternoon nap. Vincent wasn't home. A tiny stray orange cat I named Nibley had joined our household, appearing a couple of months earlier meowing for food. She was fast asleep on the couch, curled up in a tight ball. I fought the urge to curl up with her.

The red light on the answering machine blinked rhythmically.

"Not an emergency," I muttered hopefully and pressed the play button.

"Doc, this is Sherman Jenson," the message started, and already I knew there was trouble. I could hear the strained tone of Sherman's voice. He was a calm guy who moved at the pace of a cold bumblebee, not much troubled by anything, but today he sounded agitated.

"That cow that Doc Hadley worked on yesterday, with the leg abscess? She's bleeding bad from that leg, and she's down in the alleyway." That meant she had fallen and couldn't get up. A down cow was an emergency.

The gray sleepiness of the day evaporated, and my mind clicked into doctor mode, running through a list of the potential diagnoses, equipment I would need, fastest route to the Sherman dairy.

"Can you come, Doc? Hope you get this message. I called Doc Hadley and left a message on his phone too."

Sherman's farm was just out of town, thank God, not a hundred miles away in Idaho.

"Lee," I yelled, "grab a surgical pack. We've got an emergency."

The white Ramcharger roared to life. I backed down the dirt driveway too fast, hit the pavement and jerked the truck around. The rain and wind picked up, the windshield wipers swished back and forth on top speed.

"Damn," I said. "Ron told me about this cow." I wiped the inside of the fogged-up windshield with my sleeve.

"She had a nasty leg abscess he lanced yesterday. Got a quart of pus out of it, then bandaged it up." I was driving too fast through town. Although our local police were extremely vigilant about speeders, they never stopped me because they recognized the truck and knew that if I was driving over the speed limit, one of their friends somewhere had an animal that needed something fast.

I wheeled into the long gravel driveway. The rain came down hard, pelting the ground. I grabbed my raincoat and jumped out of the truck. No one was around. Except for the rain, it was so quiet I thought for a minute that maybe I had misunderstood the message. I saw Sherman's team of Clydesdale horses out in the back pasture, their shiny black backs glistening, grazing in the rain. When I had first met Sherman, he told Ron that he wasn't keen on a woman working on his cows, but he would give me a chance.

"Just don't let her near my pulling horses," he told Ron. Sherman was protective of his prize Clydesdale team. They had taken second place in the state fair the previous year. Ron had been Sherman's vet for a couple of years, and they bonded over a shared love of horses and mules. I'd been doing preg checks and vaccinations for Sherman for a couple of months, and I thought I had earned his trust, but only for his dairy cows. I was intimidated by the Clydesdales and happy to accommodate Sherman's wishes to not mess with them.

I heard a shout around back of the barn. Sherman had seen us pull in.

"Out back, Doc!" he yelled. "I got some hot water." Farmers always thought that no matter the emergency, a pail of hot water was required.

I grabbed my bag, and Lee and I pounded around the barn. There was the cow, on her side, in a pool of blood that looked as big as a pond, thrashing her legs. She made a loud, guttural call of panic and distress. It's a sound of pain and hopelessness that makes it hard to think straight. Sherman had a halter on her, which was a blessing, because he could at least keep hold of her head. Her thrashing had stirred up a froth of blood, manure, cow pee, and mud. Dairy cows are handled enough that they are usually docile, but when injured, all bets are off. These Holstein cows can give a well-placed kick that can easily break the knees of someone standing in the wrong place.

Sherman, his son Jared, and another farmhand all turned to me with looks of trust and relief when I walked up. They were sure that now that the doctor, even if it was only the lady cow vet, was here, everything would be fine. Their panic and worry flowed into me, and my job was to absorb it and radiate calm, while my brain was roiling, trying to figure out what to do.

"Sherman, what happened?"

"Don't know, Doc. Yesterday, Doc Hadley lanced that abscess on her leg, bandaged it up nice, and gave her a big shot of penicillin. We thought she was all fixed up. Just now, I drove by on the tractor when I saw her out here, shaking that leg like crazy."

"Okay, let's get a rope around the back legs. Each of you hold one." Thank God we had three big men to help.

The cow lay on her side. I waded through the blood, looped a rope around the top leg, high up on the hock and handed the long end to Jared, who, like his dad, was built solid and strong.

"Stretch that leg back so I can get at the bottom one," I told him. I could see that the top leg was not the source of the problem.

"So anyway, Doc," Sherman said, "I saw that bandage fly off with one of those shakes, and I didn't think much of it. But then later, when I came up to start getting the girls in for milking, there she was, down, with blood everywhere."

Lee was trying to get the other back leg secured, but the cow, seriously upset with the restraint, was throwing herself around so violently it was hard to get hold of it. We were drenched, splattered with blood and mud.

I tried to focus on what might have happened, realizing that although Ron had cleaned out the abscess, there might still be an infection in that leg. If it had been as big an abscess as he said, then it could have been deep enough to eat away the artery that runs down the leg as the main source of blood for the foot. The only thing that could account for so much blood loss was an arterial bleed, and the only thing that would stop it was tying off the bleeding artery. But if that was the major source of blood to the foot, then would tying off result in loss of the foot?

Lee and Sherman struggled to restrain the spurting leg while Jared held the other leg and the farmhand pulled on the halter. I tried to remember the vascular anatomy, but no matter how hard I tried to shut out the chaos, I couldn't remember exactly how the nerve, artery, and vein course down the leg.

My patient gave a huge bellow and stopped struggling for a minute. Because she was stretched out between ropes, I got a good look at the wound. I clamped my hand over the skin and muscle above the abscess and the flow of blood stopped, as long as I kept a heavy pressure. At least now I felt the situation was somewhat under control.

"Okay," I said, lowering my voice to sound strong and confident. "Here's what I am going to do." Dr. Hammel's advice popped into my head. "You never stop being afraid, you just stop showing it." I smiled.

"A bandage won't help here. I think the infection has eaten into an artery. I'm going to have to suture it up. Then we'll put her in the hospital stall and bed it real deep with straw, and I think she'll be okay."

A parallel voice in my head kept saying, "Yeah, she'll be okay if her foot doesn't fall off for lack of circulation when I tie off the main artery, or if she doesn't get septic from this open wound being drenched with manure, or if the infection doesn't spread up her leg."

In the rain and gloom, I couldn't see the damn artery. When I took the pressure off above the wound, the squirting fountain of blood obscured it.

"Lee," I said, "come on over here and put pressure on this leg. Right here."

"Okay," I said. "Now we're in business!" Even with the bleeding slowed, the artery was too deep to see. I'd just have to suture by feel and accept that I could be tying off other tissue, including nerve and muscle. This would not be pretty. When I sunk the needle into the wound, the cow kicked so violently I fell back hard on my butt, and the suture, needle, and needle holder went flying into the muck.

"Hold those ropes!" I yelled. "I can't tie off this blood vessel unless you guys can keep her from kicking!"

The cow was bellowing even louder, rolling her big white eyes back in her head, as if she was dying. I knew she wasn't—a cow that can kick that hard has plenty of life in her. But she had lost so much blood, and was already down, I thought it might kill her if I tried to tranquilize her. I rinsed off the suture and needle holder in the hot water, which was no longer hot, and splashed some alcohol on it, knowing that a little alcohol couldn't possibly clean this level of contamination.

"Let's give it another try."

I didn't think this was going to work. Maybe if the cow lost enough blood, then we could restrain her better. But if that happened, she might die of shock, and then who cared about a suture around her leg artery? My raincoat was useless. Water rolled down my neck, soaked through to my butt from the fall. I felt it pool inside my rubber boots.

Lee looked at me and winked. Crazy or not, we were giving it a shot. That cleared my head, and I approached the leg again, this time from a different angle. But before I touched her with the needle, she seemed to sense me coming. She jerked in several directions all at once with her neck and both back legs, knocking all three rope holders off their feet and throwing me into the muck, flat on my back.

This was a Mormon town and a Mormon dairy. All my clients were Mormon. They did not swear. They did not take the Lord's name in vain. The very worst thing that I had heard in Cache Valley, when someone was really peeved, was "Well, my heck!" That was considered extreme.

But I had grown up in upstate New York. My parents were atheists. When my father hit his thumb with a hammer, it was common for him to say, "Son of a bitch!" or "Goddamn it to hell." Now I say "Fuck!" in the same way, but back then, no one used the "F" word. In the world of Mormons, I put a filter on my bad language, careful to respect their cultural aversion to swearing. But when I was kicked, covered in blood and manure and drenched to the bone, thrown into the muck for a second time by a very large Holstein cow whose life I was trying to save, something snapped.

"Goddamn it, you bitch!" I screamed. "Goddamn it to hell, just hold still! I'm trying to help you!"

"Son of a bitch!" I spat out. "Jesus Christ!"

Lee's mouth opened and shut.

"Hold those ropes!" I yelled. "Put your back into it, for God's sake, we're going to get it this time." Lee grabbed the leg again and held on for dear life, putting pressure on the wound. I dunked the needle holder in the dirty water and leaned hard against the cow's belly.

I braced myself against the taut leg and sank the needle deep in the general area of the artery. The cow, by now weaker and feeling the determination of the rope holders, tried a perfunctory struggle and grunted while I tightened the suture and tied it off. Not sure

I had tied what I needed, I did another big suture and tied that one off too.

There was a solemn silence among the men.

"Okay, Lee, take the pressure off." This was the moment—had I tied off the artery? For all I knew, I could have tied muscle, or worse, a nerve. Lee gingerly released her grip on the leg. The bleeding had stopped. I felt a flood of relief.

"Keep those ropes tight!" I ordered. "Lee, can you go up to the milking parlor and get a new pail of hot water? Bring a towel too."

There was no sense in suturing the skin—the wound was hopelessly contaminated and needed drainage. The cow seemed thoroughly spent, and it was a relief to hear her moan instead of bellow. The four of us stood silently in the rain, the men looking at their boots, waiting for Lee to come back with the hot water.

When the bandage was finally on, with several layers of stretchy bright purple bandage material holding rolls of cotton in place, the real test came.

"Let her back legs go, very slowly. One at a time." Sherman went around to her head, clicked his tongue and murmured gently to her. I could tell by the way her ears perked up that she was okay. She scrambled to her feet and shook her head.

I wanted to get her out of the rain before the bandage soaked through. She limped up the alleyway, Sherman guiding her, hand on her halter. In the hospital stall bedded with straw, she went straight to the water tank and put her big nose in, sucking down gallons. Losing that much blood made her thirsty, and I was relieved to see her drinking. By now it was almost dark. Sherman switched on the barn lights.

There is something about a stall freshly bedded with deep dry golden straw, fragrant alfalfa in the feed bin, and a big old cow that inevitably calmed me down. I slumped down in the corner, on the bad leg side of the cow, and watched for signs of any blood soaking through the bandage.

A lot of bad things could happen over the next forty-eight hours: fulminating infection, sepsis, gangrene of that leg if it didn't get

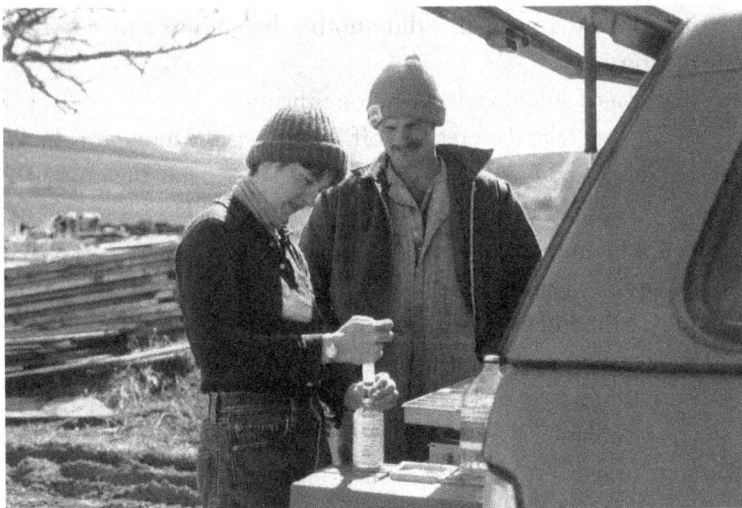

Linda and Greg Mauchley. Linda is mixing up an antibiotic solution for Greg to administer as a follow-
up treatment for some coughing calves.

enough blood supply, nerve damage if I had caught a nerve in
the suture. But for these few minutes—while Lee cleaned up our
equipment, the sun went down, and the barn grew dark—with
blood matted in my hair, my clothes soaked to the skin, and rain
still pelleting down, everything was just fine.

"I think she'll be okay for now," I said to Sherman. "I'll come
by in the morning to check on her." I got up, stiff and sore from
the struggle. "And you come out here around ten o'clock tonight
and have a look for any bleeding. If you see any, even a little on
the bandage, you call me."

"Sure will," he said. "I usually come out late to check on the
team." Sherman loved his Clydesdales.

Lee was in the driver's seat, truck idling, when I came out, and
we headed home. She smiled—she had lived in Logan longer than
I had and knew what was happening.

The next morning, we arrived at Greg Mauchley's dairy just
after milking. He came out to greet the truck.

"Morning, Doc!" he crowed. Greg had finally decided the lady cow vet knew her stuff, after seeing me in action for a year. We had developed a friendship of sorts, which included him ribbing me for not going to church and suggesting that if I would just read that Book of Mormon he gave me, I could be saved and go to heaven.

"I heard you used some pretty salty language over at the Jensons' yesterday," he grinned. "Swore up a blue streak, Sherman told me. Wish I was there to hear it."

Yes, and it wasn't just Greg. Every single client within a hundred miles had gotten a call from someone who had gotten a call from someone else. That lady cow vet has quite a mouth on her. You should have heard her let loose. Well, my heck!

CHAPTER 27

THE LOW-CEILING BARN WAS FREEZING in the early January morning. The cow lay on her side on a bed of straw, and I sat beside her. We stared at each other. This was my third visit to the Mickelson dairy in a week, and I still had no idea what to do with her. The warm breath from her nostrils condensed in the cold, making puffs of white while she chewed her cud rhythmically. A wedge of fragrant alfalfa hay was piled next to her head, along with a tub of water, so she could eat and drink when she liked. She hadn't gotten up in a week. Three or four times a day, Riley Mickelson came with one of his sons and shifted her thousand-pound bulk from one side to the other so she would get some circulation in the leg under her heavy body.

She wasn't the typical milk fever cow, weak from lack of calcium. She had a mild case of mastitis and seemed to be getting better with treatment, but after milking one day, she stumbled and fell in the alleyway. Riley used his tractor and a skid to drag her into the barn, bedded her deep with hay, and called Dr. Hadley to give her calcium, to no effect. She hadn't broken a bone. We had pushed and prodded her, but she just looked at us with her big brown cow eyes, not making any effort to rise.

She might have a selenium deficiency known as white muscle disease, sometimes seen in older cattle, so I had given her an injection of selenium. Blood work had not provided any clues. In the meantime, each day, each hour that she lay with so much weight on her leg muscles made it less likely she would get up.

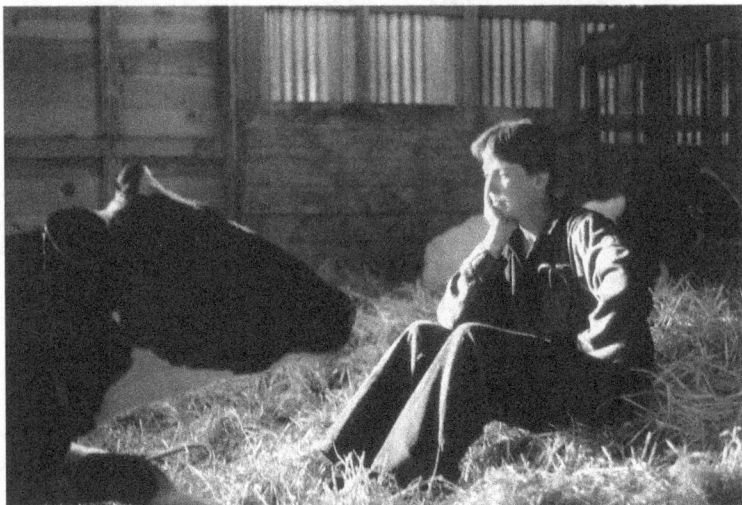

Linda with the down cow, Pinky, on the Mickelson dairy in Idaho.

Riley came in the barn, squatted down in the hay next to me, and patted his cow on the neck. He'd been doing his best, keeping her on a deep bed of straw and moving her from side to side. The cow's name was Pinky, and his affection for her was clear.

"Doc," he said, "I think it's about time we threw in the towel." Riley's family had milked cows for decades, and he and his brother Lawrence worked the family farm, with their father, Harris, for many years. I'd been a vet for only a year and a half.

"She doesn't look too bad."

"Her milk is drying up," he said. He was right. She was costing him time and money and would for another year even if she did, by some miracle, stand up. He would have to feed her for all that time until she freshened and he could sell her milk again.

"It's a shame, but I think she's a goner. I've got three of her daughters in the herd. Pinky was a terrific milker," he said, shaking his head. He reached over and gave her neck another pat. The Mickelsons were dairy royalty. They had been farming in Grace, Idaho, for generations and were known for having the highest-producing Holsteins in the state. Big, kind men, gentle with the cows, with dozens of children, they worked seven days a week, up before dawn for the morning milking, out in the alfalfa fields to hay in the heat of summer, chopping ice from the watering troughs in the winter. You would never find a pile of broken-down equipment or a sloppy barn at a Mickelson dairy. Manure was scraped, stalls were bedded with straw or sawdust. The milking parlor was scrubbed to a shine after each milking. When Ron had signed the Mickelson dairies up for his herd health program, it was a sign to the entire valley that Ron knew what he was doing.

I wasn't willing to give up, but I knew Riley was right. I had failed to figure out what was wrong with this cow, and the longer I puzzled, the less likely the cow would ever get up. I had dug through my old vet school notes, talked to Ron about possibilities, and reached a dead end. I felt sick.

A calico barn cat snuck into the stall and sat in the patch of sunlight washing her face with her paw. Riley and I were silent. He picked up a piece of alfalfa hay and broke it into small pieces, watching me.

"You did the best you could, Doc," he said. That "Doc" was such a sign of respect, it broke my heart. I didn't feel I deserved it.

"Not good enough," I said, standing up and brushing straw from my jeans. "Just not good enough."

❖

A few weeks later, I was back at the Mauchley dairy, deep into a C-section. Now that both twins were delivered, I felt more confident. Two live calves and the mother doing fine, surgery almost done. Spring was on its way, I could feel it in the breeze across the broad alfalfa fields, the sun a little brighter, the days a bit longer.

"Hey Doc, she's up already!" I glanced over at Greg toweling off the first little heifer twin. His coveralls, like mine, were covered in stringy, clear mucus and streaked with blood. Broad back bent over the second calf, he held her hips to steady her. She shook her head so hard her wet ears flapped against her cheeks. I loved that sound.

Mama cow shifted her weight and groaned. I had closed the

two-foot incision in her uterus. Lee handed me a new curved needle threaded with thick black catgut to suture the first two layers of muscle. The final layer would be the skin, needle-dulling tough.

"What do you figure?" Lee said. "Another hour?" She looked as tired as I felt, her blonde braids flecked with straw, coveralls smeared with blood.

"God, I hope not. I'm beat. I need coffee."

She sighed. "I need a shower."

My sutures went in neatly, and the gaping incision was closing nicely. The barn was chilly, and I heard the sputtering of the calves' breath clearing the remaining mucus from their noses. Greg was toweling off the second twin. The first one stumbled in the hay, trying out her new legs.

"Hey Doc," Lee said quietly. "Did you feel that?"

"What?"

"The cow—she . . . maybe," Lee trailed off.

"What?" I was busy suturing the incision.

"Just thought I felt a thump, on her side here," Lee said, her blonde eyebrows drawn together, concentrating.

"Boy, you must be tired." I grabbed another bite of muscle in the needle and pulled the suture taut.

Greg looked over from the other side of the stall. "Everything okay, ladies?" He was working on twin number two, rubbing her briskly with a dirty towel. Since last year, when he hadn't trusted me to do surgery on a cow with a twisted stomach, I had been at his dairy a couple times a month, treating calves with scours, cows with cystic ovaries, toxic mastitis cases, stitching up wounds. He had finally gotten comfortable with the fact that I was a real vet.

"Yeah," I yelled. "Almost done here. Can you get us another bucket of hot water?"

"Coming right up." He threw the towel on the hay bedding and headed to the deep sink.

My fingers cramped from tying suture knots, my feet were numb from standing on the cold cement floor in my rubber boots, and my shoulders ached. Lee had arrived at my house at three a.m., and we rode from Logan through the dark countryside across the

Utah border, up the Valley to Idaho to help Greg with the calving. Thank God it was the beginning of summer, and the sun came up early. Greg was one of the best dairymen around and one of my best clients. When he called and said he couldn't get these twins out, I knew it was going to be a C-section.

Damn. I felt it, too. A thump. Exactly that. Like the cow's heart had given an extra hard beat.

"You feel that?" Lee said, leaning on the cow. We stared at each other.

"Oh . . . my . . . God." I had almost finished closing the incision, and I was pretty sure another calf was in there thumping around. "Triplets?" I'd never heard of a Holstein having triplets.

Lee watched me slide my hand back through the part of the incision that was still open. I put the flat of my hand against the side of the huge uterus and, oh yes indeed, I could feel a small, kicking foot.

"Greg!" I yelled. "You ever hear of a Holstein having triplets?"

My dairymen had so many years of experience, going back generations, that their knowledge almost always trumped my book learning.

"Ha! Doc, don't fool around with me." He set the bucket down hard, hot water sloshing. "Holsteins don't have triplets."

"This one does."

"Well, my heck! Triplets?" He stared at me, took off his cap and scratched his head. "I've never had triplets born here. Are you sure?"

For Greg, "my heck" is big deal profanity. He came over and peered into the incision. There was nothing to see yet, but he knew I was serious—I was pulling out the uterine sutures I'd just finished placing.

"Goll darn. I'll be!" More high dudgeon for a Mormon. Greg was not an excitable guy, and I smiled to see him so worked up. He went to wash his hands so he could pull out calf number three.

I glanced at Lee, who was bustling around cleaning up our equipment. "How's mom doing?" She laid her hand on the cow's rump and looked her over. "Seems fine, Doc. Want me to get the calcium?"

"No, you stay here to help Greg. We can get some calcium into her once I get this little one out."

The calf's slippery butt end was facing up, so I had to reach up to my shoulder, deep inside the cow's uterus, to find a front foot and then a second one. Greg came back and grabbed the feet.

"The head is turned—let me get the neck straight," I said. The small calf's neck was bent back toward its flank, and I felt for the mouth, slipping my fingers in so I could hold the jaw to straighten the neck toward the uterine incision.

"That's it, Greg, pull!"

Ten seconds later, all eighty pounds of calf were up and out, on the pile of straw behind the cow. He was already shaking his head and sneezing mucus out his nose. I stared at him in disbelief—I had delivered triplets.

"Okay, Lee," I said, "Now let's get that calcium into her. Greg, you take care of the little guy." Greg lifted the little calf into his arms and carried him over to a bed in the clean straw.

"Diane!" Greg yelled to his wife. "Diane, come see! We got us triplets!" Greg kneeled in the straw and rubbed the dark, wet hair of calf number three. "Call the *Idaho News*—they're gonna want to know about this."

Using the large scalpel, I trimmed off the now ragged edges of the cow's uterine incision so that I could sew it up again cleanly. Lee and I looked at each other across the mama cow's back and grinned.

The uterus, the muscle and skin stitched together, some calcium in her veins and antibiotics in her muscle, poor mother was finally free to lie down and rest.

"Triplets, bless her heart." I patted the old girl on her rump. Greg busied himself with feeding all three calves colostrum out of plastic bottles with nipples. The sisters were sucking fine, but little brother was turning his head away.

"Diane, here, you work on this little guy," Greg said, handing the bottle to his wife, who had come back to the barn to help out.

The sun had been up for an hour. Lee and I needed to clean up. We had a forty-five-minute drive back down the valley before starting on the day's calls, which were already piling up on the answering machine. But we took our time, laughing and patting the three newborns on their wet heads. We speculated about who

IDAHO NEWS

Harris Mickelson

An interesting and very unusual incident took place at the Gregory Mauchley dairy last week.

A four-year-old cow of Greg's was in labor but did not seem to deliver. So the vet, Linda Rhodes V.M.D., was called. She made and examination and decided the case was complete torsion (or twisted uterus). A cesarean section was performed by Dr. Rhodes, assisted by Ms. Lee McEnery, Veterinary Technician, and Greg. Three live calves were taken from the cow, two heifers and one bull. All calves lived and the cow is doing very well also.

I have only known this to happen once before in this area. Clark Mickelson had a cow deliver triplets many years ago. Two of them lived and the other one died.

Some Idaho dairymen will be classifying their herds around the middle of April. It is reported that Utah will be done earlier.

William Lupo will be the inspector. Mr. Lupo has been classifier in some parts of Idaho previously.

The herd owners who requested special classification, put in for a May classification.

The new building being erected on the Franklin County Fairgrounds at Preston, Idaho is coming along on schedule. All concrete work is done and erection of the main building is under way.

Catalogues for the Quality Corner Sale are now available. Contact President Laurence D. Mickelson, Star Rt. Box 379, or phone 208-427-6642, Grace, Idaho.

Catalogues for the Idaho State Sale are also being done and will be here in ample time for the sale.

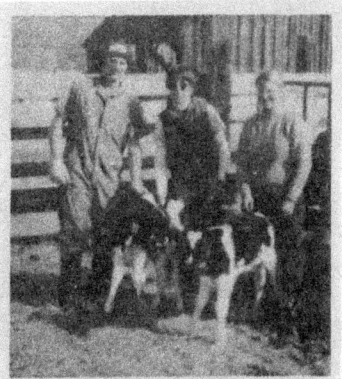

In the picture, left to right, are Gregory Mauchley owner of cow and triplet calves, taken cesarean. Linda Rhodes V.M.D. who did the work assisted by Ms. Lee McEnery, Veterinary Technician.

Article in the *Idaho News*, written by Harris Mickelson, announcing Linda's delivery of triplets by C-section.

might win the blue ribbon in the heifer category at the Idaho State Fair this year. Greg had won it last year with a lovely almost all-white Holstein heifer named Sparkle.

Harris Mickelson, Riley's dad and another client of ours, whose dairy was just over the ridge, served as the local reporter for the *Idaho News*, and he was on the way with his camera. A clear blue sky glowed, a fresh breeze full of sweet alfalfa and silage blew in, and Greg stood with an arm around Diane, enjoying the sight of his three new calves standing shakily by their mother. These triplets were going to make him famous in Gem Valley and maybe beyond, by golly, and darn it if it wasn't the lady cow vet who delivered them.

CHAPTER 28

ON A STILL, CLEAR MORNING in May, the snow-topped Wasatch Mountains glowing pink with dawn light, I went out to the truck to check my supplies for the day's calls. In a couple of days, it would be my thirty-first birthday. Maybe Ron would give me the day off.

Vincent was asleep. The breeze brought the fragrance of new grass up the valley. The crescent moon shone clear in the dawn sky. I took a deep breath of pine-scented mountain air and stretched. Lee's car was approaching—count on her to be on time. A trail of dust followed her little yellow car up the dirt road.

"Got the list?" she asked.

"Yeah, just now off the answering machine. Not too bad a day."

"Who's first?"

"The Jensons' dairy, just out of town. Then we head north. All routine stuff."

"Thank God for that! After yesterday, we need a quiet day."

The day before, we had left at dawn and didn't get home until after eight p.m. A couple of emergencies had stretched the day to the breaking point. I ducked into the house and brought out a couple of blueberry muffins to share.

"Not homemade, but not too bad," I said, mouth full.

We drove down the valley to Main Street, past the Straw Ibis café, not yet open, and then north to the Jensons' place. They milked about a hundred and fifty cows, and ten were on this morning's list for a pregnancy check, plus a couple of problem cows that had not settled—if they didn't get pregnant soon, they'd be sent to slaughter.

I wanted to check the cow whose leg I had stitched up, swearing in the rain, a while ago.

I didn't see Sherman Jenson's team of Clydesdale pulling horses in the pasture where they usually grazed. Maybe they were in the barn for the blacksmith. Such giant horses that worked as a team to pull a sled with ever-increasing weights needed regular shoeing. Sherman Jenson had told Doc Hadley that it might be okay for that lady vet to work on his cows, but he wanted Ron to take care of his precious pulling horses. Ron owned a bunch of mules and liked equine work, so I was happy to have him handle the routine worming, vaccinations, and occasional muscle sprain of the Clydesdale team.

The gravel drive crunched beneath our tires on the way up to the milking parlor. I noticed a couple of extra pickup trucks down by the horse barn. Jared heard us and waved. Jared, Sherman's son, worked with the big horses, harnessed to the pulling sled, building stamina and muscle.

"Doc!" he yelled. "Got a problem. Come on down. Bring the truck."

"What's up? Where's your dad?" I asked. Jared was young, and if there was a real emergency with the horses, I needed his dad.

"Looks like there was a big fight in here last night." Jared pulled off his cap and scratched his head. "The new gelding's hurt pretty bad, Doc."

I grabbed my kit. "Let's take a look."

In the dim barn I saw the stall had been shattered, thick two-by-eight planks splintered to toothpicks. The young Clydesdale faced the corner, trembling. His teammate, the older black gelding, was now out in the pasture.

"What happened?"

"Blackie and Clyde were our best pulling team, and you know, Clyde died of the colic a few months back." Jared talked faster than his normal Utah drawl.

"We got this here young fella, Gus, last week, and we thought Blackie was getting used to him."

The two horses were housed next to each other before they had time to become friends, and Blackie had beat up Gus—badly. Gus had a huge hoof-shaped tear in the muscle of his massive butt, with a flap the size of a dinner plate hanging down, exposing the underlying muscles. He had ragged, bleeding scratches on his shoulder and more on his front leg.

"Where's your dad?" I asked again. I was going to need Sherman's horse skills to help me with this giant. Gus was tall enough I could walk under his belly without having to duck too far. Like his potential pulling partner, Blackie, Gus wore the horseshoes of a pulling team horse—heavy iron made to gouge into the earth for traction, matching the large size of the wound in his butt. Blackie had cornered Gus and kicked him mercilessly.

Sherman's pickup came down the hill. His brown lace-up boots were caked with mud from the alfalfa field, his gray baseball cap pushed back on his head, matching the gray of his hair. Solid, Mormon to the core, big hands, six-feet-plus tall with a gentle demeanor that made him a good match with his pulling horses.

"Hi Doc! I went looking for Doc Hadley, couldn't find him. We got us a real bad situation."

"I can see that."

"I know you aren't much for horse work," he said, stepping into the stall and murmuring reassurance to Gus, patting his neck.

"You're right about that," I said. He was reluctant to let the lady cow vet near his prize pulling horses, but right now, he didn't have much of a choice.

Sherman stood close to Gus, gently rubbed his muzzle, and talked softly into his ear. There was no way I was getting near that wound without Gus being sedated. My go-to drug was fast acting and usually sedated an animal for about thirty minutes. To calculate the dose, I guessed Gus's weight to be about eighteen hundred pounds.

"Okay, Sherman. I've gotta give him an IV. Can you hold his head?"

I moved slowly into the stall. Gus's tail started to switch.

"I got him, Doc. You go ahead."

I leaned into the left side of the horse's neck. His head towered over mine. The jugular vein stood out in his massive neck. I eased the needle in, pulled back the plunger, saw a stream of purplish blood run into the syringe, and slowly injected the dose.

Within a minute after I'd administered the sedative, Gus should have slowly lowered his head toward the ground and become calm and sleepy. But he just turned his head in my direction, put his ears back, and stared at me with his wide brown eyes. The barn was quiet except for some flies buzzing. I looked at Lee. We both knew the drug should have taken effect by now.

"I'll check the expiration date," she said.

We waited. It was now mid-morning, and the sun was hot. The barn smelled of alfalfa hay and warm oats. Barn cats sat in the corners, licking their paws. Gus needed stitches in his butt, and to put them in, I had to stand directly behind him in the line of fire of two hind legs, big as lampposts.

"I hate horse work," I said under my breath to Lee.

"I know," she said. We waited for the sedative to kick in.

Sherman looked at me. He held Gus by the halter and ran his big hand over the horse's soft muzzle. "Maybe you can give him a little more?" he said.

"I can't. If I give him too much, he'll go down and could hurt himself. I think it's not working because he is so worked up."

"Poor guy is shaken up for sure," Sherman said, patting Gus's neck.

I busied myself with my stethoscope, checked his heart, his breathing, ran my hands down his legs, thinking I should have done a physical before administering the sedative. What if he had some internal injuries? Lee brought a couple of bottles of lidocaine and a large syringe from the truck. She was right, I would have to do the sutures using a local anesthetic.

Gus's tail switched nervously. He was a gelding, about three years old, shiny brown coat with a white patch on his left front foot. His magnificent mane cascaded over his massive neck. He was built to pull—well muscled and beautifully proportioned.

"Here's the plan." I put some iodine in the bucket of hot water John brought. "Sherman, you hold onto Gus's halter and get that twitch on him. You're the best man with a twitch. Get him thinking about his nose so he's not thinking about killing me." I looked around the stall, planning an escape route should Gus explode.

"Sure Doc, I got him."

"I'm gonna stand right up close to his butt, close as I can so he can't wind up a kick," I said. My best escape strategy seemed to be to duck under the shattered boards dividing the stalls. Gus could probably charge through them, but they would delay him enough that I could get away. Sherman stroked the big gelding's nose and gently pulled a section of his nose and lip through the twitch chain and twisted it, not too hard but hard enough to draw Gus's attention.

"This big needle is going right into his wound," I said, holding up the thick steel needle attached to a sixty-cc syringe. "He's not going to like it one bit, but once I get it in, I'll inject this stuff that will numb him up, and he shouldn't feel much of anything after that."

I leaned on Gus's left side with my body tight against his flank and slowly slid along and around his hip until my chest was pressed directly against his huge rear end. I stood as close as I could, feeling the heat of his body through my coveralls. From this position, his kick could throw me across the barn, but he couldn't wind up a kick that would break my legs. His rear end was taller than me, and the ragged, bloody, oozing wound was at the level of my face.

When Lee handed me the lidocaine-filled syringe, needle attached, I almost dropped it my hands shook so badly. A hush came over the barn. I took a deep breath and plunged the needle directly into the wound, deep, and simultaneously pushed on the plunger.

Gus jumped straight up. He levitated several inches, and the full weight of his body came directly down on all four hooves, the crash shaking the barn. I heard Sherman suck in a sharp breath. I kept my eyes on the wound and my hand on the syringe, with the needle still embedded in Gus's butt. Thank God it hadn't flown into the hay. Then—silence. I waited to the count of sixty for the first bit of lidocaine to take effect.

Gus dropped his head down and started to look like a sedated horse, maybe the sedative was starting to kick in after all. I took another deep breath, my heart pounding like a jackhammer. I backed the needle out half an inch, hoping that the area was numb enough that Gus wouldn't feel it while I infused the lidocaine around the circumference of the wound to numb it. Sweat pooled on the small of my back.

Still pressed up close to Gus's butt, I reached back to Lee. She handed me a bottle of saline to pour over the wound, cleaning it up as best I could. The sturdy, thick brown catgut suture material was the heaviest gauge I had in the truck. I placed individual sutures, about thirty of them. Gus shifted his weight from one foot to the other. Suturing is hard when your hands are shaking.

"Doc, you okay back there?" Sherman said. He had been holding Gus's head the whole time and didn't have a view of the action.

"Almost done," I said.

Lee pulled up a big dose of penicillin. "Okay for me to give this?"

"Sure, use his left neck muscle."

"Okay, Sherman, you can let him go." I had backed away and was more than a leg distance from Gus. He loosened the twitch and leaned his face against Gus's, whispering to him it was all over and everything was going to be all right. Those pulling horses were Sherman's big babies.

"Let's see what you did, Doc" he said, walking around to look at Gus's rear end. "Mighty neat job. You think he'll be okay?"

"Should be fine, as long as you can keep him away from Blackie."

Gus moved toward the water trough, lowered his head, and took a long drink. Good sign. He looked steadier on his feet. The trembling had stopped. His butt would be numb for a few hours, so at least he would feel a bit better now. None of his other scrapes needed suturing.

"He's going to be one sore guy for a couple of weeks," I said. "Call me if you see any discharge from that wound, or if he runs a fever."

"Nice job, Doc," Jared said. Sherman nodded.

From these two guys, this was high praise.

"I'll come back next week to check on him. The sutures won't need to be removed—they'll absorb on their own. Try and keep him clean—plenty of straw in the stall."

Lee washed up and had the equipment back in the truck when I climbed behind the wheel, and we smiled at each other. It was the beginning of another long day.

CHAPTER 29

THE ROAD NORTH TO IDAHO snaked through an endless valley of wide rolling hills and pastures, surrounded by the Wasatch Mountains running north to south. To the west, Old Baldy Peak and Oxford Mountain, to the east, Cottonwood and Sedgwick Peaks, with ranges of lower unnamed high hills fading away in the distance. The land was an expanse of grass, with narrow river washes full of cottonwoods shaking silver in the summer breeze. I'd been working for Ron for just over a year, and I never got tired of this drive through the empty countryside.

Crae Fuhriman's dairy was in Downy, a small town near Lava Hot Springs, Idaho, ninety miles north of Logan, population around four hundred. The natural hot springs had been made into a public bathing area where you could soak year-round. The southeast corner of Idaho was part of our practice area, and Crae's dairy was the farthest north we went. Crae milked four hundred cows, one of our biggest dairies, and he grew alfalfa on a couple hundred acres of fertile soil. His hay was second to none, rich leafy blue green, smelling of summer and milk. He cut and baled it, then shipped it on huge semi-trucks, rectangular piles stacked high, covered with brown tarps, barreling west to California for dairies in the Central Valley.

Twice a month it was my turn to drive up to Lava Hot Springs. If I scheduled things right and there were no emergencies, Crae's dairy would be my last stop, and I could be done early enough in the afternoon to bathe in the hot springs, where I soaked the

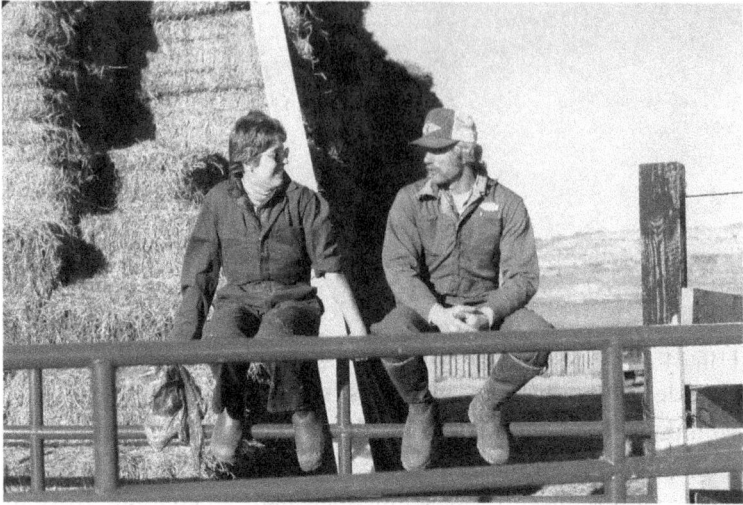

Linda and Crae Fuhriman after completing preg checks
in Downey, Idaho. (Notice Linda's rolled-up left sleeve—
she did rectals with her left hand so she could write her
findings in the medical record with her right.)

manure out from under my fingernails, leaning my head back in
the steamy water to replace the cow smell with sulfur-tinged steam.

Crae had invested in barns and equipment that made my job
easier. A large roomy pole barn was open on both sides, with a
cement walkway down the center, and metal stanchions on either
side. When I arrived, the feed truck was just finishing its drive
down the center of the barn, spilling out silage or hay. Crae waved
at me and shut the big machine off. He walked down the center
aisle while the cows came up to the stanchions and pushed their
big black-and-white heads through the metal bars to feed. When
he got to the end of the barn, he pushed a lever to trip a locking
mechanism that caught all the cows' heads at once, lined up in a
row. It was a wonderful alternative to chasing the cows around a
muddy pasture or holding pen to corral the one that I needed to
examine.

One scorched summer day, I pulled my dusty truck up at the Fuhriman dairy around noon. A couple of hundred Holstein cows lay around the barn on their sawdust beds, udders filling up for the afternoon milking, chewing their cuds, jaws moving rhythmically. I strolled around, enjoying a quiet few minutes before Crae came out and we had to get to work. The still air smelled of warm alfalfa hay and cow manure. One heifer wandered around, restless. I guessed she was in heat. I walked closer to the fence, hoping to see her ear tag number so I could let Crae know she was ready to breed.

On the far side of the enclosure, a large black cow, a white spot on her forehead, lay on her right side, head flat on the ground, her left side swollen like a tight balloon the size of a fifty-gallon drum. She wasn't moving. I stared for half a breath and then ran flat out to my truck. She was bloated, and bloat can kill a cow within minutes. Gas builds up in the rumen, the first of four stomachs, to an internal pressure that can stop the heart. From the back of my truck, I grabbed the rumen trocar, an instrument that has a sharp point and a hollow center, designed to plunge into the side of the cow, through skin and muscle, and penetrate the rumen to let the gas escape. I ran back to the stanchions and vaulted over. A sharp edge of jagged metal on the stanchion ripped a deep gash on the inside of my left arm. Blood spurted over my coveralls and ran down my arm. I ignored it and hit the ground on the cow side of the fence, running.

At the sound of me pounding toward her, that damn cow jerked her head up, gave a tremendous, sonorous belch, and scrambled to her feet. Blood dripped down my arm onto my hand, unnecessary rumen trocar at the ready. She turned her heavy head toward me and stared, like she was thinking, *What was all that fuss about?* I clamped my dirty hand over my gash and slunk back to the truck. I could have clapped my hands or yelled from my side of the fence, and she would have sat up and burped out that gas. Instead, I had to play superwoman. Thank God no one was around to witness the vet being so stupid.

Crae drove up in his pickup after I managed to bandage myself with a roll of cotton and some bright purple bandage wrap.

"How's it going, Doc?" he said, looking at the messy bandage on my left arm, the blood on my coveralls and the trail of blood from the stanchions to the truck.

I shrugged. "Just a little nick from the fence."

"You okay for preg checks?"

"Sure, let's get going."

"You sure you don't want to get that checked? Maybe you need stitches."

"I'm fine," I said. "But you can lug my gear box if you would."

In a couple of hours, after we finished the preg checks and as I was washing up in the milking parlor, Crae could see I was favoring my arm.

"Better get that looked at before you drive home."

"I'll be fine," I winced as I peeled off my dirty coveralls.

Crae shook his head. "Up to you, Doc."

By the time I got on the road, my whole arm was throbbing. Pulling off to the side of the deserted road, ten miles out of Lava Springs, I unwound the wrap and pulled the blood-soaked cotton off the tear. It was worse than I thought—angry and red, right down to the muscle. Crae was right—it needed stitches.

I felt so alone, sitting on the side of the road near the Idaho-Utah border, my arm a bloody mess. I was tired of the constant pressure I put on myself to be perfect, to never make a mistake, to feel that if I screwed up, it reflected on all women trying to do this job in the future. I could have laughed at how silly I must have looked, rushing to save a cow that just needed to belch. Instead, I was telling myself how stupid I was. A constant crushing responsibility not to screw up had worn me down, more than I had realized.

❖

By the time I got to the emergency room in Logan, it was late. The only doctor on duty was a young intern. He looked like a high school kid dressed up to play a Mormon doctor.

"How'd this happen?" he asked. The ragged skin was cut in a wedge about an inch long. He picked at it with a tweezer. I winced.

"Cut it on a metal fence at a dairy."

"That means a tetanus shot," he said. "I'll put a few stiches in and get you started on antibiotics."

I lay back and gasped when he swabbed the wound with iodine, the pain bringing tears to my eyes. I felt the sting of a needle and the cool lidocaine numbing my arm. I sat up to watch him stitch. His hands shook when he sank the curved suture needle into the edge of the wound and pulled the skin taut over the gash. I realized that I had probably stitched up dozens more wounds than he had. Human medical interns don't get a fraction of the surgical experience a veterinarian does.

"Don't put so much tension on the suture," I said. He looked up at me, frowned and started the second stitch, pulling it just as tight.

"It's gonna leave a scar."

"Oh, so now you're the doctor?" he sneered. "I know what I'm doing."

I lay back down and sighed, too tired to argue. Yes, I thought, I am now a doctor. Just a stupid one who tried to save a cow that didn't need saving.

On the inside of my left arm, I still have an inch-long, bleached white scar with little scar dots on each side marking where the doctor had pulled the suture too tight.

PART FOUR

Breaking Point

CHAPTER 30

NIBLEY, THE LITTLE ORANGE TIGER cat I had taken in when she showed up thin as a stick on my front porch, was skittish, afraid of the rattle of dry leaves, afraid of the distant sound of a dog barking, afraid of people. Over the past year, she had put on weight, but she was not a cuddler. The warm waterbed was a comfort to her, and she slept against my leg but jumped down the moment I moved to pet her.

I'm not sure what frightened her enough to climb the tall oak tree in our front yard, and when I realized she was up there, I was more worried than if it had been Logan, who was wise to the ways of the world and would have been down in a few hours for dinner. When Nibley didn't come down overnight, I had trouble sleeping, and by late afternoon the next day, I was wild with worry. When I looked at her so high up in the tree, she cried a loud meow, staring down at me. I felt awful not helping her.

It was an early August Sunday, warm cloudless blue sky, clear mountain air. Vincent's friend, a drummer named Dave I hadn't met before, was setting up his drum set in the living room. There was some talk of forming a new band, maybe a bass player would join them later. Dave, torn t-shirt, smelling of weed, drove his beat-up pickup up to the house and unloaded his drums. I could hear the snap of the snare drum, the clamor of the cymbals. Then I heard the familiar sounds of Vincent's electric guitar tuning up.

I went into the living room. "Nibley's still in the tree," I said. Vincent shrugged and twisted the E string peg. "She needs help getting down."

Vincent plucked the string, and I heard the pitch rise as he turned the peg, his ear to the guitar.

"Can you give me a hand to try and get her down before you start rehearsing?"

"How?"

"I think the neighbors have a ladder."

Vincent sighed, looked at Dave and shrugged. He didn't bother to try and convince me that Nibley would come down on her own. "I guess so," he said, putting his guitar down on the couch.

Dave jumped up. "I'll give you a hand."

I watched the two of them walk down the driveway to the neighbors', while I tried once more to lure Nibley with the aroma of a newly opened can of tuna fish. The borrowed ladder was the kind painters use, aluminum with a ratchet mechanism so that the ladder could extend as high as a second-story window. Dave propped it against the tree.

"Great, perfect." It was tall enough to reach the branch Nibley was perched on. I watched Vincent crank it higher, clacking a metallic *clank* each foot it rose. Poor Nibley huddled against the trunk, terrified. We stood back and looked up.

"Take my backpack. You can stuff her into it." Looking back, I wonder why it was Vincent that climbed the ladder, because of course I could climb a ladder just as well as he could. Why I asked for his help instead of climbing that ladder myself, I don't remember.

"Don't need it. I can grab her," he said. He grasped the edges of the aluminum ladder and started to climb.

"At least put on something with long sleeves so she won't scratch you," I said. He wore his heavy black work boots, jeans and an old white t-shirt.

He ignored me—he just wanted to get this over with. It was a simple job. The ladder rested against the sturdy branch where tiny Nibley perched wide eyed.

Dave said, "Watch out for those wires." I looked up, shading my eyes, at a utility pole about a dozen feet from the aluminum ladder. The electrical wires running from the pole to our house ran through the branches of the old oak. The bright sun glared in the cloudless blue sky.

Nibley, meowing her small meow, inched toward Vincent, watching him climb. She could see he was almost up to her branch. As shy as she was, she was eager to come down. Dave and I stood back to get a good view of the rescue operation. A bright, brittle, yellow flash cut the sky, we heard a vicious hiss, and Vincent fell back off the ladder, arms outstretched. Time slowed. He hit the ground hard with a sound that made me nauseous. In two steps, I was on my knees cradling his head. He seized while I tried to open his mouth, thinking I needed to get his tongue out of his airway. My heart pounded.

My fault, my fault, rang in my head.

Dave must have called 911. Vincent was limp. I couldn't tell if his heart had stopped. I started CPR. From a long way away, I heard the ambulance siren coming in slow motion and then faster down the driveway, billows of dust behind. They strapped Vincent on a gurney, loaded him in the ambulance, and gestured for me to jump in the back. I moaned quietly, rocking back and forth on the seat. I watched the paramedics cut Vincent's pants up the front and strip them off. The faint sickening odor of charred flesh rose from Vincent's leg.

The paramedics had checked—his heart was beating. Vincent, completely limp, eyes closed, had an oxygen mask over his nose and mouth. I heard them say his blood pressure was low. They started an IV. I stared at my thumb, dripping blood on the floor, and idly wondered why I was bleeding. The siren screamed in and out of focus on the short drive through the quiet streets of Logan. The waiting ER team took over, lifting Vincent out and rolling him away; the EMTs bustled inside. I was alone.

After a while, the driver came back to close the back doors of the ambulance and saw me sitting there. "Honey, go on inside," he said kindly, and I did, my thumb dripping a line of red across the floor. A bored woman looked up from the reception desk.

"You can sit over there," she said. So I sat.

In a few minutes, a young man in green scrubs came out the back of the ER and looked around the waiting room. Maybe there was someone else there, but I didn't see them. Tears streamed down my face, my nose dripped.

"You with the guy who just came in?" he said. I nodded.

"Tell me what happened."

"He fell," I sobbed. "The wire must have touched his head, and he fell."

The doctor sat down next to me. "How far was the fall?"

"I don't know—about twenty feet? When he hit the ground, I thought he was having a seizure." I stared at the floor and swallowed. "I tried to get his mouth open, but his teeth were clenched."

I put my hand on the doctor's arm. "Is he alive?" My voice seemed way too loud—was I yelling?

"Yes, he's alive." He looked straight at me, saw my bleeding thumb and took my hand in his. "What happened here?"

I looked down and saw my entire thumbnail was gone—only a raw surface, oozing blood.

"He must have bit it when you tried to open his mouth."

What had he said about Vincent? He's alive, but barely? Brain dead? Crippled?

"Let's get a bandage on that. When was the last time you had a tetanus shot?"

Someone handed me a tissue for my tears, but I wrapped it around my thumb, its touch stinging the raw bleeding flesh. It didn't matter. The woman from the front desk came over.

"Dr. Rhodes? There's a call for you."

"For me?" Nothing made sense. Who would call me at the hospital? And how did that ER woman know my name? She stretched the black cord over her desk and held out the handset. I put it to my ear.

"Yes?"

"Dr. Rhodes, this is Bishop Johannson. We heard about the accident."

I wiped my nose on the back of my hand. "Who?"

"Bishop Johannson. I'm the bishop in Logan. We're sending someone down to the emergency room to sit with you."

It dawned on me that he was the bishop of the Church of the Latter-day Saints—the Mormons. What was he saying?

"We'll bring some food—you probably haven't eaten." I shook my head no, looking at the phone. No, I hadn't eaten.

"And Sister Jessy will bring a blanket. You might be in that waiting room a while."

"What?" I said, nothing registering.

"You don't need to say anything. We'll be there to help you. Goodbye, Dr. Rhodes. Someone will be there soon." I heard the dial tone, handed the phone back to the woman, and sat on the cold plastic chair. When the doctor came back with a few things in his hand, he sat down next to me and laid them out on the table. A stainless steel bowl with some water. Some bandages.

Who is that for? I thought.

"Just put your thumb in the water. It'll soak off the tissue."

I did what he told me. Soon I had a proper bandage on my thumb. I leaned back in the chair.

The LDS ladies arrived with chicken salad in a Tupperware bowl, a white roll, and a small carton of milk in a cloth sack. They didn't ask me what happened, left the food on the table next to my chair, and sat down a few chairs away. One pulled out her knitting. Another doctor pushed out the swinging doors and walked directly over to me.

"Are you the wife?"

"Yes."

"Your husband is unconscious but stable. He sustained some pretty bad burns where the electric current blasted out his foot. He'll likely lose two toes, maybe three." I was seated, looking up at him. He was telling me that Vincent was alive.

"The current also left a deep wound on his ankle and some nasty burns on his scalp." Wounds, burns. But his brain—what about his brain?

"Can you tell me exactly what happened?" the doctor said. "It'll help us figure out a prognosis." I stood up, pushed the hair off my forehead, and took a deep breath. The doctor waited.

"My cat was in a tree. My husband got a ladder from the neighbors." I could see the LDS women leaning in to hear. The waiting room was quiet. I felt like I was shouting.

"He put the ladder against the tree and climbed up. I was looking up at him and the cat. Then I heard a hiss, and he fell."

"So, it was his head that touched the electrical wire first?"

"Yes, probably. I guess so. He fell a long way." I was crying again.

"And how did he land?"

"On his back. I thought he was having a seizure."

"Good he didn't land on his head." I couldn't ask if he would be okay. I knew he would never be okay. "He's still unconscious. We can't evaluate his mental condition," he said. I nodded. No answer to the question I most wanted—needed—answered.

"Is he paralyzed?"

"Oh, no, his reflexes are intact. His spinal cord wasn't damaged." The doctor's pager went off. He gave me a pat on the shoulder.

"You stay right here. They'll help you with anything you need." he said, gesturing to the LDS women. I found the bathroom, peed, and washed my face. It wasn't easy. I couldn't use my left hand with the thumb bandaged up. I sat on the toilet and stared at my sneakers spattered with blood. It took a minute to realize it was my blood. Vincent hadn't been bleeding.

Fried, I thought. His wounds wouldn't bleed because they were cauterized by the high-tension current that knocked him off the ladder. I remembered the smell of charred flesh in the ambulance. In the waiting room, a blanket and pillow had been arranged on the only couch. I was alone with the LDS women. I thought about my cats. Nibley—what happened to Nibley? And Logan would need some food.

"I need to get home to feed my cats," I said to the nearest LDS woman. She was an older lady, maybe sixty, with graying hair and a kind smile. "I need a ride," I said.

She stood up and put her arm around my shoulder.

"No dear, you need to stay here with your husband." The younger woman, a girl really, stared at me.

"The bishop sent someone up to your house. The door was wide open when you left. We fed the cats and closed up the house." I looked at her, dumbfounded. She said "cats," so somehow Nibley must have made it home.

"How did you know I had cats to feed?"

"The bishop takes care of things like that when there's an emergency. We'll take turns feeding your cats."

"And feeding you," the older woman said. She nudged me to the chair next to the chicken salad.

"You need to eat. Heaven knows how long you might have to be here."

I don't remember eating, or laying down or falling asleep, but I remember the doctor shaking my shoulder. When I opened my eyes, the waiting room was bustling, and the sun was up.

"He's stable. There's nothing new to tell you, except his blood pressure is better."

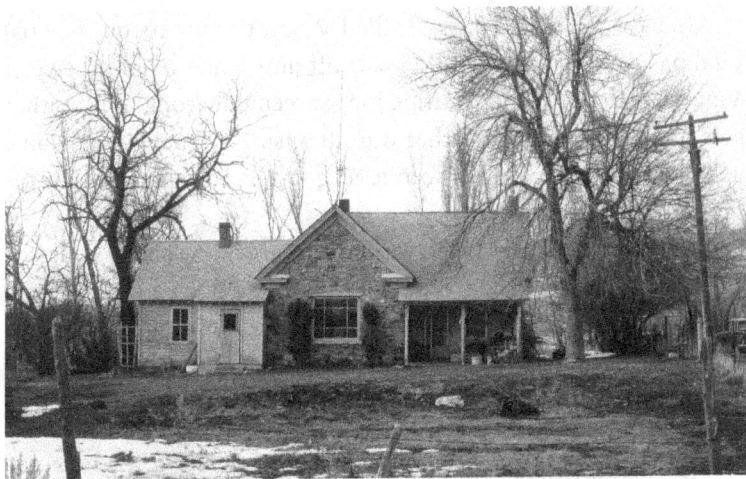

Stone house in Logan. The telephone pole on the
right is the one that electrocuted Vincent.

"Okay, thanks," I said, groggy with sleep. I needed coffee, but there was none here, and it was one thing I couldn't request from the LDS ladies.

Two new LDS women were there, and one came shyly over to me. Her face was scrubbed, hair in a neat braid and her yellow dress looked recently pressed, contrasting with my disheveled state. I had left the house in jeans and a t-shirt, my shoes were spattered with blood, and I badly needed a shower.

"We brought you a hairbrush, a toothbrush, and some tooth-paste," she said, holding out a paper sack.

"The nursing staff said you can go in the back and use their dressing room if you need to."

❖

For the next seventy-two hours, I wore the same clothes, ate LDS food, with LDS women as mostly silent companions, and waited for Vincent to wake up. I slept, read stupid magazines about celebrities I had never heard of, paced around outside the hospital. Late at night, I cried. Mostly I stared at the floor, replaying the accident in a horrible vivid loop.

After twenty-four hours, I called Vincent's parents on the hospital pay phone. I thought I'd put it off until I had reliable news of Vincent's prognosis but waiting longer seemed wrong. His mother screamed and cried; his father was all business. They would come as soon as they could. I ran out of quarters and had to sign off before we could make plans.

I missed my cats. And who was taking care of the cows? I guessed Ron, but I hadn't heard from him. My thumb pulsed with pain on my left hand—my palpating hand. On the morning of the third day, before sunrise, the waiting room dim and empty, a different doctor came through the swinging doors.

"Dr. Rhodes?" he said. "Your husband is awake!"

I jumped up. "Awake?"

"Yes, you can see him now."

My hair was matted, and I smelled of three days of cold sweat. "Is he okay?"

In the intensive care unit, Vincent leaned on pillows propped against the back of the bed. He wore a white hospital gown with small blue flowers on it. An IV dripped pain medication into a vein in his hand. Bandaged and elevated on a large pillow, his right foot looked huge. His dark curly hair was in disarray, part of his scalp shaved and bandaged. I stood in the doorway watching him try to focus his eyes on me.

"You okay?"

He nodded.

"They got me drugged," he said, his words slurred.

The doctor confirmed, "Heavy pain meds for his burns. We think he suffered a concussion when he fell."

Vincent patted the side of his bed. "Come over here," he said. I carefully put my arms around him, my head on his shoulder. We lay together, breathing.

"Okay, Dr. Rhodes, he needs to rest," the doctor said. I patted Vincent on the shoulder. He was already asleep. I could go home for a bit. The LDS ladies drove me.

My fridge was full of casseroles, my vegetable garden was watered, my cats were fed, even the grass was mowed. Nibley acted as if nothing had happened. A note on the kitchen counter from Ron said he would cover the practice for a couple of weeks. After a hot shower, clean jeans, and a fresh T-shirt, I wolfed down bites of tuna casserole, cold, standing in the kitchen with the refrigerator door open. Logan and Nibley rubbed my legs. They stared up at me and both licked a little tuna I offered with my finger.

"Gotta go, cats," I said, petting each of their heads.

I drove back to the hospital, where I spent my days for the next few weeks, arriving each day before dawn. I wanted to know all the details of Vincent's care and prognosis, and there were already insurance forms to fill out. At home in the evenings, there were phone calls from my parents, my sister, Vincent's family. Everyone was worried, but no one came to help. I had fitful dreams full of darkness.

❖

The doctors couldn't predict how Vincent would recover. Getting electrocuted by head-butting a high-tension wire and falling twenty feet to the ground was not a common accident. But the doctors knew they needed to manage the pain, and Vincent was suffering. His second and third toes had to be amputated—no live tissue was left. The wound that tunneled down to the tendons in his ankle was worrying, and the daily debriding was so painful he had to be on morphine. His mental condition was hard to assess.

Vincent's parents couldn't afford the flight to Utah. They stayed in Rochester and talked to Vincent on the phone. He made an effort to sound normal to them, and they agreed they would come later, maybe when he was out of the hospital and they could get cheaper airfares, or better yet, he could come home. For his parents, Vincent's home was their house.

Sometimes Vincent was lucid, sometimes he was silent and confused. We didn't talk about the accident. He didn't ask about Nibley. I sat in an awful plastic chair in his hospital room, reading anything I could distract myself with, while he slept, which was most of the time.

CHAPTER 31

I DROVE VINCENT HOME A few weeks later. Walking was painful. The waterbed was a good place for him to start healing—warm, yielding. He only wanted to sleep. I bought crutches. We tried to figure out a daily routine, but disrupted by pain, everything was in flux.

Vincent lost a lot of weight, his appetite gone. He felt weak and helpless. There wasn't much I could do for the pain, but I did everything else I could think of. Meals, laundry, endless insurance claims, cozy fires in the woodstove. September mountain nights near the Wasatch Mountains were cold.

The LDS ladies came now and then to bring another casserole. They picked up their empty dishes and talked about the weather. The bishop had said that even though I wasn't a member of the church, I helped all the dairy farmers in the valley, and that meant they should help me. Grateful for their care, I began to understand why people converted to the Mormon faith.

The worst were Vincent's bandage changes. Twice a day, sterile gloves, silver sulfadiazine cream for healing the burned tissue, wet and dry strips of sterile gauze, wrapped with just the right amount of pressure to keep the oozing down but not so much to cut off good blood flow. I thought back to that Thanksgiving when I'd been in charge of Josie's bandage changes, long before I had any idea what I was doing. Now I had the knowledge, but it was no easier. Pain was ever present. Vincent had to take a narcotic before the bandage change, but no matter how careful I was, it hurt. Three times a week I drove him to the hospital for a debriding procedure, which was more painful than the bandage changes. Debriding removed dead tissue from the wounds to encourage healing. Vincent's foot and ankle soaked in hot swirling water to soften the tissue, and then his doctor picked dead bits out of the wounds with a tweezer. Sometimes he pressed dry gauze on the wound and tore it off, along with blackened chunks of skin and muscle. After several weeks, when all the dead tissue from the third-degree burn was finally removed, the doctor did a large skin graft on Vincent's ankle. The pain wore Vincent down, and it wore me down to see him suffer.

After two weeks of taking care of Vincent nonstop, Ron called.

"Gotta get back in the saddle, Doc," he said cheerfully. "I need you."

"Getting back in the barn would be great," I said. Truthfully, I wanted to start being the lady cow vet again, tired of pain and paperwork. Plus, we needed the money. "Can't do those sixteen-hour workdays, Ron."

"Can't you hire a nurse or something?"

"On the salary you're paying me?" My tone was light, but geez, Ron.

❖

I completed Vincent's bandage change before I left for work in the morning and after returning in the early evening—it took almost an hour. The cows were a welcome relief. Just getting out of the house of pain lifted my mood. The golden quaking aspens stood out against the rich blue sky, the mountains already dusted in brilliant white snow. On the way out of town, I drove by the Jenson farm. Sherman was out in the field with the Clydesdale team harnessed to a pulling sled, their magnificent muscles straining. Looked like Gus and Blackie had made peace with each other. Sherman saw my truck and waved, making me remember how good it felt to be in the barn with the cows where I could do some good and the dairymen would thank me daily. Driving home after dropping Lee off, the sun was a red ball touching the horizon in the west when I pulled my truck into the driveway.

The house was freezing. Vincent was under the covers in the heated waterbed, and the bedroom window was broken.

"Threw my shoe at it," he said. I looked at the broken window, jagged glass scattered on the bedroom floor.

"Why?" I asked. He shrugged. It was me he was angry at, I thought—he blamed me for asking him to go up that ladder.

Something was happening. Vincent, normally calm and silent, was angry. Flashes now and then, a vicious curse at someone who bumped his crutches on the way into the hospital, shouting at the radio news. It worried me, this gentle man, lashing out. Maybe some company during the day would help. I asked a friend who worked at the university to stop in and check on Vincent during her lunch hour. She and Vincent got along well, and I think he liked the visits. Most of the day he slept—it was the drugs. He didn't play his guitar or mandolin, nor did he read a book. Life was on hold for him, all his energy going to healing.

At the next appointment, while the doctor was checking if the skin graft was healing properly, I found the emergency room doctor who had bandaged my thumb. He shook my hand and then took a look at my thumb and smiled. "Looks like the nail is growing back nicely," he said. "How's your husband?"

"He's angry," I said. "It worries me." We were walking briskly down a long hall—he was on his way to another emergency.

"Typical of a concussion victim. We see it a lot. Unexplained and out-of-character anger."

"Really?" I said, feeling relieved that it might be a medical phenomenon.

"I wouldn't worry unless he turns it on himself."

"On himself?"

"Yeah, suicidal. Sometimes these concussion patients get suicidal." I stopped, and he stopped too.

"But I'm not there all day. I have to be at work."

The doctor looked at me. "You better get some help," he said.

Maybe I could believe that Vincent didn't hate me for asking him to get Nibley out of the tree. Maybe he had a medical condition that made him angry and possibly suicidal. Either way, his anger vibrated just under the surface, and it scared me. He was too hot for me to handle. I wasn't worried that he would hurt me but that he might hurt himself. I called his brother Frank that night, after Vincent was asleep.

"I need you to get out here," I said. "This week. Now."

"Why, is he worse?" Frank said.

"Not physically. His foot's healing slowly." I explained what the doctor had said about the concussion and Vincent's anger. Neither Frank nor his wife, Kathleen, had full-time jobs in Ithaca. She made silver jewelry and was a part-time pastry chef, he was a musician. They had the flexibility to come help, but no money for a flight. I agreed to cover the airfare, and Frank said they would come that week.

❖

I hadn't realized how exhausted and overwhelmed I was until Frank and Kathleen moved into our little house in September. We had lived together in a commune in Hop Bottom, Pennsylvania, back in 1973, the year before I went to vet school, and Vincent had lived with them in the Freeville commune during the years I went to Philly to study. They had left the commune a few years ago. Neither had changed much. Kathleen still had lovely long strawberry blonde hair and a goofy smile. She wore ankle-length paisley skirts, filmy cotton blouses, and jewelry made from shells and feathers. Frank was full of rhythm and grins when he had a fiddle in his hands. He and Vincent were clearly brothers, with similar features and mannerisms. Neither of them talked much.

Frank and Kathy settled into the back bedroom. Kathleen took over the cooking. Frank encouraged Vincent to play his guitar, which felt like a minor miracle. The house was comfortable with them in it. I went to work knowing that Vincent had company, healthy food, and music to cheer him up.

When I arrived home from work, the three of them sat in the living room, Kathleen and Frank on the couch, Vincent in the rocking chair with his damaged foot on a pillow on the footstool, the house warmed by a wood fire. I stripped off my filthy coveralls, threw them in the washer, and took a hot shower. Drying off, I hummed a little tune, looked at myself in the mirror and smiled. I could feel happy again, if just a little. Kathleen had a pot of spaghetti boiling, and an apple pie in the oven. I slept better. I worked hard. I tried not to worry.

Summer was over, the days shortened, dark when I got home from work. Vincent moved better on his crutches. His doctors tapered off his pain meds. Frank and Kathleen had been with us about three weeks, our routine worked well. I was up early to give Vincent his pain meds and do the bandage change. He'd drift back to sleep, and I could leave and not worry—I knew Kathleen would get him breakfast. In the evenings, Vincent was more alert, and he played guitar accompanied by Frank on the fiddle. The music helped him forget the pain for a bit—I was happy to see him smile. I drifted off to sleep with a backdrop of music and the aroma of baked goods wafting through the little house.

One evening, I was surprised when, after Vincent was asleep, Kathleen and Frank came into the living room where I was getting ready to bed down on the couch. Vincent had the waterbed to himself ever since he came home from the hospital. Kathleen threaded a long pink ribbon she used as a hair tie between her fingers, not looking at me.

"We have a couple of things we need to talk about," she started.

"Can it wait until morning?" I asked. I was propped up on a couch pillow, hoping to get a minute to look through *The New Yorker* before I fell asleep. "Long day today and another long day tomorrow."

She shook her head. "We need to go home." Need to go home? I sat up straighter. "But Vincent can't be on his own."

"We think he can," she said, looking at Frank, who looked down at the floor. "He's much better now," she said, firmly. "We need to go back to Ithaca. We've been here almost a month."

I went into the kitchen, sat at the table, and stared at the wall. Logan followed me in, thinking he might get more dinner. I put my head down, forehead on the cold table and took a couple of deep breaths. My body was beat—too many early mornings, too many late-night emergencies, pushing too many cows around, all while worrying about Vincent every moment. Logan rubbed my legs. I reached down to pet him. The living room was silent when I walked back in. Kathleen was rocking in the rocking chair. Frank stood next to her, his hand on her shoulder.

"I need to get back to my job," she said. "The longer I'm gone, the less work they'll have for me."

"But Kathleen," I pleaded, "What am I going to do?" Frank shifted from foot to foot, chewing his fingernail. "You guys have been great, but I need help. Before you leave, can we arrange for someone else to come? Maybe Anthony? Your parents?" I said, turning to Frank.

He shrugged. "You can ask."

"And here is the bill for the airfare—round trip," Kathleen said, handing me a receipt. I looked at it—the amount was astronomical.

"Yeah," she said. "It was expensive, getting those tickets on short notice."

I had just enough savings to cover it, after paying the deductible for the medical bills not covered by the health insurance that I had thankfully forced on Vincent.

Their food, a place for them to stay, gas for the car, and the outrageously expensive flight was the deal for three weeks of their help. Now they were leaving without offering to help me solve the problem of Vincent's care and my full-time job. How would I pay all the bills, including my student loan payment, if I had to quit my job to stay home? I barely had enough money in the bank to cover their airfare. I gulped back tears. A private nurse would have cost more, I told myself, trying to calm down, trying not to be furious. After all that communal living, this is where things ended up: back in our nuclear family corners, looking out for our own interests, being willing to help but only up to a point.

"Can you at least give me a week or so to figure something out?"

"Sure, of course," Frank jumped in before Kathleen could say no. She shot him a look. "What about your parents?" Kathleen asked. "Can't they come out?"

I couldn't believe she would ask.

"My mother has terminal breast cancer. They have enough to worry about," I said. She put her hand to her mouth, her eyes blinking rapidly. She had forgotten about my mother's illness. They went to bed, and my thoughts raced. My sister, Anne? Her daughter, Satya, was now in grammar school, so spending time in Utah wasn't possible. Vincent's older sister? Doubtful she would be able to get away. She had several children and a strict husband. Vincent's parents? Very unlikely. Vincent's father ran a small family grocery store, and his mother took care of Vincent's disabled sister. And Vincent's youngest brother, Anthony, wasn't the caregiver type. He liked to smoke dope, play music, and write poetry. I couldn't picture him helping much, but he could at least play music with Vincent and keep him company. I'd have to do the cooking and everything else, but Vincent wouldn't be alone all day if Anthony came. I would call him in the morning. Exhausted, I lay down on the couch and turned off the light.

Wouldn't it be nice, I thought, *if Kathleen and Frank had called Anthony and arranged to have him come out before they told me they were leaving? "Linda, we have to go, but we made sure you will have the help you need," they could have said. "Don't worry, we will help you every step of the way."*

Nice, I thought drowsily. *That would be so nice.*

❖

I was out the door at three a.m. for a calving emergency and made it home to shower and change Vincent's bandage before my real day started. After my shower, Kathleen and Frank sat in the kitchen drinking coffee and looked like they wanted to talk, but I ran out the door pretending I had another emergency. I just wasn't in the mood. By the time I made it home after work, it was late on the East Coast—too late to call Anthony.

CHAPTER 32

By October, most of the leaves had fallen off the big oaks and rattled around the front yard. The chill wind whipped silver clouds over the Wasatch Mountains. Frost was thick on the windows in the dim Sunday morning dawn. It was hard to believe it had been less than a month since the accident. Everyone slept in. Both cats curled up beside me on the living room couch. The house smelled of wood smoke from the fire that died out overnight. I watched the sun come up behind the clouds, laying on my couch bed, looking out the frosty picture window at the graying ominous sky. In a few days, I'd be back to being Vincent's sole caregiver. I was dreading it.

The phone ring jerked me to my feet, scattering the cats.

Damn, I thought. *A Sunday emergency call.*

"Dr. Rhodes," I answered, my professional voice, still in my jammies.

"Hi Linda." It was Dusty.

"Hi! Dusty! It's early!" I realized if it was early in Utah, it was really early in California.

"I know," he said. Something felt wrong. I could hear him breathing.

"It's Josie," Dusty said. "She's in the hospital."

I dragged the phone cord back to the couch and sat, pulling the blanket over my legs. "Why, what happened?"

"She broke her leg getting out of bed," he said.

"Where are you?" I asked, trying to picture the early morning emergency.

"Pasadena Hospital emergency room," he said. "And they broke her arm."

"What? Who?"

"The nurse when she arrived. Josie told him to be careful, but he didn't listen," Dusty was speaking softly, his voice strained.

"What happened?"

"He grabbed her arm, and it broke when he lifted her out of the wheelchair," Dusty said, his voice angry. "It's her cancer. It spread to her bones."

"Oh my God," I said. I hadn't realized how far her breast cancer had advanced. I had been so involved in my own drama with Vincent.

"Is she okay?" I said stupidly. Of course, she was not okay. She was dying of breast cancer.

❖

I don't know how I expected the final days of Josie's illness to go. I hadn't had time to think about it. Dusty had shielded me from knowing how fast things had progressed. If the metastatic tumors were so far advanced that her bones were breaking, I knew her time was short.

"She's okay for now. They're casting her leg and her arm."

"And good pain medication, I hope."

"She's resting. She didn't want me to call you."

"I'm coming," I said, swinging my legs down from the couch and standing up.

"No, no, you can't," Dusty said. "What about Vincent?"

"Goddamn it!" I yelled, waking everyone up and frightening Nibley, who ran and hid under the couch. "I'm coming to Altadena."

Vincent wasn't dying. My mother was.

"You do what you feel is right," Dusty said. This is what he always said, but I could hear the relief in his voice. He needed someone who could understand medical jargon, someone who could talk to the intimidating oncologists. He needed his doctor daughter, doctor of many species.

"Dusty, you go and be with Josie. I'll get there as soon as I can."

"Okay," he said, and added, "Love you," which broke my heart.

I felt my legs wobble and sunk down on the couch. My hands trembled; my brain raced in a thousand directions. Panic, sorrow, fear, the weight of all of it, heavy and dark. My mother, only fifty-eight years old.

Not now, not now.

❖

Kathleen and Frank were in the kitchen and heard enough to get the gist. Vincent was awake but silent, rocking on the waterbed waves. I lay down on the couch and pulled the blanket up to my chin, staring out at the clouds. I was going. To hell with my job, to hell with Kathleen and Frank. Now they would have to take charge. I was getting on the next plane to Pasadena.

Fierce, angry love for my mother coursed through my body, blasting out my fingertips and toes, girding for battle with death, knowing I would lose. This most important fight, the fight for a "good death" for Josie, as best we could manage. Kathleen and Frank whispered in the kitchen. Vincent hobbled to the bathroom. I pulled on my jeans and sweatshirt, found the yellow pages directory, and looked up airline phone numbers. Kathleen came into the living room and wordlessly handed me a mug of hot coffee.

When Vincent came out of the bathroom, we gathered in the kitchen.

"Josie is dying, and I am going to Altadena to be with her and Dusty. I don't know when I will be back."

Vincent nodded and reached across the table. I gripped his hand—it was cold.

Kathleen started to say, "But what about . . ." when Frank cut her off. "We'll figure something out."

Frank drove me two hours to the Salt Lake City airport that afternoon, after I called Ron to tell him I was leaving, quitting my job, actually. I didn't want to be the lady cow vet anymore.

Ron wouldn't hear of it. "Just take a leave of absence," he said.

My focus was elsewhere—not on cows, work, money, Vincent and his problems. The life I had built in Utah seemed like a distant story. I would deal with all that later. I tried not to let myself know that later meant after Josie had died. By sunset, my plane took off from Salt Lake City, and I headed west, into the light, to the hardest chapter of my life.

❖

Three weeks later, the rental company wheeled the hospital bed out of the living room. Someone had gathered up the IV bags, urine-filled catheters, tubing, and soiled linen. No one cried. Dusty put a record on the phonograph, but when Mozart came on, he had to turn it off, the music too sweet for the hard month that we had been through.

Anne was there. Vincent, too, on crutches—I had pleaded with him, and he managed to come for Josie's last two days. Dusty sat in the big black leather chair, wiping his black-rimmed glasses with a white cloth handkerchief. No one was hungry. Anne and I walked through the garden to the guest room to nap, weary and drained. My eyes were heavy and wet. I couldn't remember when I had last slept.

Josie didn't want her family to deal with her body after she died. She had arranged for a cremation service that spread her ashes in the Pacific Ocean. Friends came to the house for Josie's celebration of life a few days later, and we heard stories of her kindness. Dusty drank too much of his homemade red wine and sobbed. They had been married thirty-eight years.

❖

Vincent's mother, Ida, a devout Catholic, prayed for Josie during her last days. When I told her that Josie didn't believe in heaven, Ida, with such pure faith it took my breath away, said, "Won't she be pleasantly surprised!"

CHAPTER 33

THE HOUSE FELT HOLLOW THAT winter. Losing a mother is a special kind of grief that leaves a rift in your soul. Vincent tried to comfort me, but I felt unreachable. Anne had left right after the celebration of life. She said she couldn't be in the house without Josie. She was right, it did feel bleak and joyless. Chores kept me occupied. Vincent needed to get back to his doctors, and my checking account was perilously low. Kathleen and Frank had returned to Ithaca, and neighbors were feeding Logan and Nibley. I knew we had to go back to Utah. I finished sorting the stack of insurance papers and cooked enough casseroles to keep Dusty in dinners for a week.

"And when do you and Vincent have to get back?" Dusty lowered himself into his black leather reading chair. Dusty and I had never discussed my relationship with Vincent. He and Josie didn't interfere in their daughters' marriages; they supported our choices. But when Josie came home from the hospital, she told me something, before she slipped into her final coma, that surprised me.

"I never thought Vincent was a good fit for you," she said, out of the blue one morning when I was bringing her some juice. Taken aback, I stared at her. *Why didn't you tell me that years ago?*

Dusty pointed out the back window—a flash of a turquoise hummingbird sparkled in the lemon tree. My chest inflated with a breath that turned into a sigh. "I don't want you to be alone," I said.

Dusty reached to give my knee a pat. "I'll get used to it." He took his glasses off and rubbed his eyes with both hands. I think he knew that getting me back to the cows would help with my grief. "And I have to go back to work too. Xerox has been generous with time off." Work, I realized, would be good for both of us. We had been nurses way too long.

❖

When we returned to Logan, Vincent spent his silent days in the waterbed, keeping warm. Once in a while he would get up, sit on the couch and play his mandolin or guitar, but he was still on enough pain medication that he was sleepy and depressed. Logan loved to curl up with his back pressed against Vincent's leg, purring, tail and paws curled in, and I think that gave Vincent some comfort.

Ron called as soon as he heard I was in town and asked me to come back to work. Given the fact that my loan payments were due every month, I had to say yes. Vincent no longer needed round-the-clock nursing, and I needed to get out of the house. The dairymen were happy to see me back, and at least being in the barn helped distract me from my grief.

"Sorry to hear about your mom," Greg Mauchley said. "We sure missed you."

"Thanks, Greg, that means a lot."

"Polly Ann is doing better," he said, changing the subject. I had to think a minute to realize he was talking about a cow I had treated for pneumonia before I left. "Giving almost ninety pounds a day."

"And how's that outbreak of scours in your calves?" I was glad to change the subject too.

❖

Thanksgiving passed without a celebration. I was on call but had no emergencies. I phoned Dusty and we cried, talking about how Josie was a great cook and how she loved to try new recipes. Remember the half avocados filled with chilled beef consommé? And her pies—banana cream, chocolate, lemon meringue? And her quirky table decorations—old weeds painted with gilt, or a bare tree branch with ribbons.

The start of the winter was bleak, bitter cold with sleet and ice. Ron and I alternated every other day being on call for emergencies.

It was hard, but manageable. But now, on Ron's night, the answering service was calling me.

"Dr. Rhodes, the Jensons called. They have a calving."

"It's not my on-call night. Call Dr. Hadley."

"I did, but I can't get him. His wife says he's not home."

"Well, where is he?"

"She says she doesn't know."

I went to the Jensons' and delivered the calf. The next day, I swung by Ron's house to restock my truck and wash up some surgical instruments, hoping to talk to him, but he was out on his daily rounds. I left him a note: "Call me." He didn't. Ron paid me a flat salary, nothing extra for doing emergencies. I was working more, much more, but for no additional money.

On a fiercely cold winter night, Greg Mauchley called me directly at home, not through the answering service. One of his best cows was down, high fever, cough, could I please come?

"Let me try and get Ron—it's his night."

"Linda, he's not available."

I sighed. "Did you try his house?"

Greg cleared his throat. "I'll explain when you get here."

I had to go. After all, it was Greg. We were friends.

❖

Nothing was secret in the small communities around Logan. Greg told me that various farmers had seen Ron's truck parked overnight at the house of a divorced woman in town that winter. A vet truck was hard to mistake for another pickup. Everyone knew it was Ron's truck. The next day, I didn't go to my scheduled dairy visits. Instead, I went looking for Ron. I found him eating lunch at the local diner. He waved me over. I slid into his booth, and although it was lunchtime, he was having breakfast.

"Coffee over here!" he yelled to the waitress. Ron liked to make a point that he drank coffee to annoy the Mormons.

"What the hell is up? I've been covering your emergencies, and it's getting old."

"You've heard the rumors," he said, stuffing a slice of bacon in his mouth, grinning at the same time.

"Yes, I have."

"Well, they're all true. She's great in bed." I grimaced. Ron's wife, Kay, was a friend of mine.

"Too much information. Listen, Ron, I don't much care what you do with your personal life, but I can't do emergency calls every night. Vincent is still recovering and needs a lot of care. I'm worn out."

He grinned, reached over and patted my arm. "I know, it's selfish. I can't help it, though." He winked at me. "She's so much fun!"

"Goddamn it, Ron, I don't care. Do your damn emergency calls. I'm not covering for you anymore." People turned around in their chairs to stare.

"Calm down," Ron said, reaching for my arm again. I jerked away and stood up.

"I mean it. I won't be answering the phone on your on-call nights."

I stomped out. Word of this scene would get around town pretty quickly. I wondered if Kay knew. She must, if he was staying overnight, unless he was telling Kay that he was out on emergency all night.

A week later, at one a.m. on a Tuesday morning, Ron's night on call, my phone rang. I let it ring, and it woke me up out of a dark dream, cuddled in the warmth of the waterbed. After six long rings it went silent, but I was wide awake. Then it rang again, and again, and finally I picked it up. Riley Mickelson had a sick cow. She was down, and he needed me to come right away. I could hear the desperation in his voice. He wasn't calling about a calving but about one of his best cows that was having trouble getting up.

"Can't it wait until morning?" I asked. We both knew that a cow that is down for more than a few hours might not ever get up again.

"You know it can't, Doc," he said, and I knew he was right. There were no other large animal veterinarians within a hundred miles. I swung my legs out of bed. The icy cold of the floor shocked my feet. I grabbed my robe, put on my wool socks, and went to stand by the woodstove, hoping for some heat, stretching the phone cord as far as it would go.

My chest felt crushed in, my eyes stung. I crumpled down to the floor, my legs weak and unsteady. Then I cried. I cried, right there on the phone, with Riley on the other end of the line, listening to me sob.

"Doc?" Riley said.

"I'm on my way."

The porch thermometer read ten degrees below zero. I drove into the clear dark night. Riley's place was almost an hour north up in Gem Valley, Idaho. By the time I arrived, Riley had already given her calcium. She had a high fever and a nasty mastitis, her udder red and inflamed. I told Riley to hand milk as much pus out of her teats as he could while I gave her a hefty dose of antibiotics IV, and some fluids.

"Let's see if she'll try and get up," I said. Riley leaned on her side, bracing his feet against the floor, pushing and grunting, and I pushed on her shoulder. She lumbered to her feet, unsteady but up.

Riley and I beamed at each other. "That ought to make you feel better," he said. "Always nice to finish your call with the cow on her feet."

"If you can manage to stay awake, it would sure help her if you could keep her milked out," I said, brushing straw off my coveralls.

"I'd be up in a few hours anyway for the morning milking. No sense in getting to bed now."

Home at dawn, barn dirt under my fingernails and in my hair, feet frozen, I stood in the steaming hot shower and decided I would take the day off. Ron could cover for me for a change. I was going to sleep until noon and sit by the woodstove the rest of the day.

❖

Days were short and cold, with high snowdrifts and icy roads, mountains pure white against the deep blue sky, wind frostbiting cheeks. I dressed in layers of long underwear and wool socks, mittens and thick scarves wrapped twice around my throat when I went out. Vincent didn't budge outside—his mood was pitch dark. I forgot what his smile looked like. Late one Saturday afternoon, the Wasatch Mountains dark purple in the early sunset, he took a shower, put on clean blue jeans and a checked cowboy shirt. I was reading a vet journal, sitting by the woodstove, Logan curled up on my lap, Nibley asleep on the red couch. I realized he was pulling on his coat, his blue jeans hanging from his skinny hips. This was a man who hadn't been out of the house since we came back from Altadena after my mother died. He eased his burned foot into his snow boot, and I could see the pain wrinkle his forehead.

"Where are you going?"

"There's a jam session at Dave's house." Dave was the drummer who had called 911 the day of the accident. Vincent was fiddling with his guitar case. Only in the last week had he started walking without his crutches, although he couldn't put much weight on his bad foot. The fluffy Utah snow was falling faster now, as the light faded.

"How are you going to get there?"

"I'm driving," he said, staring at me.

"You can't drive. How are you going to use the clutch?" The old pickup truck we'd bought secondhand was a stick shift, and he would need his injured foot for the clutch.

"I'll manage," he yelled. "I can't be an invalid forever!"

I watched him pull out of the long driveway. He hadn't been behind the wheel since the accident. I tried to remember when he last took his pain meds.

I heated a can of tomato soup and turned the radio to a classical station—Vivaldi, *The Four Seasons*. It was snowing harder now, the night pitch dark. I read *The New Yorker*. I petted Nibley. After a couple of hours, I thought about calling Dave's house but realized I didn't know his phone number. It was odd, being in the house alone. I went to the kitchen, then back to the bedroom, not sure what I was looking for. I settled at my desk and sorted mail, paid bills, filed stuff, anything to keep busy. When I heard the plow go by, I was relieved—at least the road would be relatively clear when

Vincent drove home. I just hoped he didn't have a beer or too much weed on top of his pain meds.

I seldom wished for a TV, but I wished for one now. I needed something to do other than worry. Finally, I settled on a thick Dickens novel but couldn't concentrate—I kept thinking I heard the truck. Logan curled up next to me on the couch, my feet stretched to the woodstove warmth. I ran my hand over his warm fur. Nibley was asleep in a tight orange ball. The wait was making me crazy. What if Vincent was off the road in a ditch? He couldn't walk for help.

When he wasn't home by midnight, I was pulling my coat on over my pajamas, thinking I would drive out to look for him, when I saw the lights of his truck coming down the driveway. I went back to the couch and pulled the blanket up, pretending to sleep. After Vincent went to bed, I stared out at the night sky, stars obscured, white with snow, the house growing colder as the fire in the woodstove died out. I was on the cusp of change. I needed the energy to move me along a path, any path, and my energy was in hibernation.

CHAPTER 34

As WINTER RECEDED, THE WILLOW buds forming, snow melting off the mountains, I could feel the earth waking up. I thought of the new lambs in the university lamb shed and how they bounced around with newborn joy. It was time to get started.

I searched the vet journals for other jobs. The few listings in upstate New York were just like the ones I had interviewed for a couple of years earlier. Low salaries, tough working conditions, and likely still an aversion to a woman veterinarian. Now, with my experience, I might have a shot at one of those positions, but I needed something new. My mother's death had changed me. Settling for a relationship that had been merely adequate wasn't enough for me anymore. I think that is why Josie told me her opinion about Vincent. She knew I was ready to move on. I thought Vincent was too.

I found a listing at a California facility in Yuba City that was putting together a business venture that combined a large dairy, a cheese-making plant, a calf-raising operation, and collecting embryos from high-value cows. The salary was $16,000 a year, a couple of thousand dollars more than Ron paid. I called that afternoon, and they agreed to a phone interview. They were pleased that I had a current California license, and I guess I must have made a good impression because the embryo-transfer people contacted a few of my dairymen to find out if the lady cow vet could actually do what she said she could. Riley Mickelson confirmed that I could do thirty-day pregnancy checks and was an expert in bovine palpation. They offered me the job starting in May. After my California job interview nightmare a couple of years ago, I was amazed at how easy it was this time. But now I had experience—and dairymen willing to testify to it.

❖

I don't think Ron was surprised when I quit. The mules leaned over the fence, and their long ears perked up watching me drive up to Ron and Kay's place in Paradise. Ron was out by the mule pen, running a hose to fill the water trough. March still felt like winter, a skim of ice on the mud around the paddock. I had finished a brutal week, with a couple of late-night emergencies. I felt light and a bit giddy. I parked my truck next to Ron's and waved. Wiping his hands on his jeans, he stood up and waved back. Wind was blowing down the canyon, picking up the smell of hay and manure from the mule pen. I felt the cold down the back of my jacket. We met at his back door, and I handed him the truck keys.

"What's this?"

"I'm done."

He threw the keys back at me, and I reflexively caught them.

"You're just tired. Take a few days off." I put the keys down on the hood of his truck.

"You can give me a ride back into town, or Kay can, when she gets home from work."

Ron opened the back door of the house. "Come on in where it's warm," he said. We went into the kitchen, leaving our muddy boots on the mat. The dogs came running, hoping for dinner. "Sit down, I'll get coffee."

"No coffee, thanks," I said, pulling out a chair to sit at the old wooden kitchen table. He reached over to pat my shoulder. I scooted my chair a few inches away, avoiding his touch.

"I'm tired. Tired of trying to work things out with you. It's your practice, you run it." He looked at me and sat down. The cats prowled around our legs. He crossed his arms behind his head, looking solemn.

"It's a two-person practice now," he said.

"Was," I said.

He uncrossed his arms and sat up straighter. "No, really, I need your help."

He needed my help. Vincent needed my help. My mother had needed my help until she died, and now my father needed it. All the dairymen needed it. We had fun, Ron and I, working together. My veterinary skills were far more advanced than they were a couple of years ago, much of it due to what Ron had taught me. Now, no one in Cache Valley was surprised to see the lady cow vet show up at their dairies. Without Ron, I might have ended up back at the Pasadena Animal Hospital, taking care of a bunch of yappy little poodles.

"Why are you smiling?" he asked.

"I owe you a lot, I really do," I said, getting up. I heard Kay's car pull into the driveway. I shrugged on my coat and reached down to pet one of the dogs. "You'll manage, Ron, you always do."

Kay poked her head in the door. "You two headed to another emergency?" She figured if we both had our trucks in the driveway, something must be wrong.

"Kay, Linda needs a ride home. She's leaving her truck here." We stood and looked at each other for a moment, feeling the finality of my quitting.

I stepped forward and held out my hand. "Thanks, Ron. I mean it."

He reached to shake my hand, his grasp firm, his face expressionless. He nodded. That was the last time I saw Dr. Ron Hadley. I heard that after his divorce, he moved up to Grace, Idaho, and shed a bunch of his less productive clients, shrinking his practice. Turns out it was a one-man practice after all.

❖

By the time it was spring, we both knew it was over. Vincent wanted to be with Frank and Anthony in Freeville playing music. His accident and Josie's death had spun me around so fast that the centrifugal force was flinging me away from my center. It seemed there was nothing left between Vincent and me except pain. We hardly looked at each other. There was no sex—he wasn't attracted to me anymore. He missed his family. He was bored, maybe still angry. I gave up trying to figure it out. Who knows? I tried not to care.

"We have to talk about California," I said, not looking at him.

He was washing the dishes, his back to me. "I know," he said, in a neutral tone. Since I had accepted the job, we had avoided talking about the future. He rinsed the last plate, dried his hands, and turned to look at me. "I've got to go back to Ithaca," he said. "It's home for me."

God, I wished I knew where home was for me. Tears pooled in the edges of my eyes. "You know I love you," I said, wiping my eyes on my sleeve.

Vincent put his arms around me and pulled me close. "I know."

❖

Riley Mickelson drove all the way from his dairy farm in Grace, Idaho, to Logan to visit me. He had talked to his brothers Lawrence and Roger, and his dad, and to Greg Mauchley, Crae Fuhriman, Terry Chatterton, and some of the other dairymen in the valley. They wanted to buy me a truck and front me the money for supplies and equipment if I would be willing to stay on and take care of their cows.

"Linda, we don't know what we'll do without you," Riley said, patting me on the shoulder. He was a grandfatherly gentleman, his hands still muscular, his bearing straight and strong.

"Riley, that means the world to me," I said. "Remember when I first showed up at your farm and all the milkers came out to the truck to stare at the lady cow vet?"

Riley chuckled. "We were kinda surprised, alright," he said.

Such a kind offer, but my time in Cache Valley was over. I needed a new direction. I owed so much to the Mickelsons. They were dairy royalty in Idaho. If they hadn't accepted me taking care of their cows, I would never have been able to practice there. But they were gracious enough to give me a chance, and a chance was all I needed.

The dairymen whose cows I had taken care of over the last few years threw me a party on a Sunday afternoon after church—ice cream, cake, and lemonade. Lee came, and dairymen's wives with piles of kids. Ron, I guess, wasn't invited. They gave me a present—one of those chains to attach to glasses so they hang around your neck when you take them off—a joking reference to the fact that I was always losing my glasses somewhere in their barns, most memorably once when a cow gulped them down with a mouthful of hay. I would miss these kind people and their beautiful cows. If ever another woman veterinarian showed up in Cache Valley, I thought she just might be welcome.

By mid-May, the loose ends had been tied. Our lease on the little stone house was up. I found a place to rent in Yuba City. My new job started June 1, 1981. The weak spring sun illuminated our drab living room with its ugly flowered wallpaper and the rag rug I had bought from a Mormon lady at the local church auction. Logan and Nibley curled up on the couch, fast asleep, their whiskers twitching with dreams of mouse hunting. Vincent wandered in from the kitchen and eased himself down next to the cats, his foot still aching from the accident.

"I want to drive back to Ithaca," he said, reaching to pet Logan. A long beat of silence. We both stared at the rag rug. "Okay with you if I take the truck?"

I nodded. The truck was a rusty relic. I hoped it would make it all the way East. I had just enough savings to buy my first new car and had my eye on a tiny Honda station wagon.

"If you aren't going to sell the Peugeot, I'll take that too," he said. "I can tow it behind the truck." That was reasonable. No one in Utah would want to buy an old, very much used French car.

"You want any of this stuff?" I asked, sweeping my arm in an arc around the living room, the furniture a shabby collection mostly from the Salvation Army. As far as I was concerned, he could have everything except the cats. They were coming with me.

"I'll take the woodstove," he said. "And maybe the waterbed if I can fit it in the truck." There wasn't much else to do—we had little money to split up, and the legality of our marriage seemed like a footnote anyway.

❖

When the pickup truck was packed and secured with a torn green canvas tarp tied down with some extra rope from my vet truck, and the Peugeot hitched up to the tow bar, Vincent leaned on the driver's-side door, his long black eyelashes lowered. He stared at the dry thistles growing weedy in the front yard. Vincent looked up, and his dark eyes gazed at me for a beat. I stepped forward, and we hugged a firm full-body hug, held a few seconds too long for me. He kissed me on my forehead. My throat tightened, and my eyes felt puffy. So much pain in that kiss.

Spring had come to the valley, and the mountains had a flush of green up to the snow line. A breeze blew down the canyon, rattling the dry grass, golden against the clear blue sky. Our old vegetable garden was a mass of weeds. Logan sat on the porch, licking his paw.

"Take it easy."

"I can use the clutch, as long as I take my pain meds."

"Don't overdo it," I said. The wound in his ankle had not fully healed. I glanced up at the utility pole by the driveway. Vincent's accident seemed a lifetime ago.

"I'm not in a hurry." He smiled a smile I hadn't seen in a long time.

"Thanks for the gas money," he said. The couple hundred dollars I had given him wasn't enough to get from Logan, Utah, to Ithaca, New York. I hoped he had enough money for the last leg of the trip. Vincent climbed into the driver's seat, slammed the door, and cranked the truck to life, engine rough and loud. He was finally headed home. The truck disappeared down the dirt driveway, dust billowing behind, and turned into Cache Valley, getting smaller. I watched, the afternoon sun in my eyes.

I thought of all my dairymen, just starting the afternoon milking. The cows will give their creamy gallons, return to their barn, munch on some alfalfa hay, and settle to chew their cuds, at peace. The dairymen too, after washing down their barns, home to roast chicken, potatoes, and apple pie, resting after a long day caring for their girls.

Instead of loss, relief washed over me, and then guilt for feeling a burden lifting. After all the caregiving I had done for my mother and Vincent, all the juggling emergencies, nursing care, insurance claims, and meals in between a punishing, physically exhausting on-call veterinary job, I now had only myself and the cats to take care of. I reached down to pet Logan. I did what I had set out to do when I first thought about becoming a large animal vet in the goat barn on the California commune, more than ten years ago. The road hadn't been easy—and it wasn't over—but I had studied hard, worked my heart out, and gained the trust of the crusty dairymen who never imagined a woman could be a veterinarian. Now, even though there were plenty of moments when I was unsure of myself, I had grown the confidence that comes from hard work, failures and successes, and showing up day after day, month after month, when almost everyone expected me to give up.

"Now it's just you, Nibley, and me," I said to Logan.

I eased down onto the stone step. Logan purred, stretched and yawned. Sunshine warmed my skin, the mountains glowed against the clear blue sky. The scent of pine and mountain sage floated on the breeze. Breathing in, I thought about how far I still had to go.

Afterword

IT'S BETTER NOW. WOMEN HAVE made tremendous strides in the veterinary profession, and, in fact, there are now more women in practice than men. In the mid-1980s, things had improved from the days when veterinary classes had just one or two women, and veterinary school admissions were nearly equal among men and women. Today, more than 80 percent of veterinary school graduates are women. Women are thriving not only in clinical veterinary work but also in leadership roles. It wasn't until 1998 that a veterinary school had a woman dean; today, there are many. Even the American Association of Bovine Practitioners, a group that has historically been made up almost exclusively of men, now has women in leadership positions.

At the time of this story, I think I was the only woman large animal veterinarian in Utah. Today, with many women in large animal practice, no one is surprised to see a woman veterinarian driving up and hopping out of the truck for a farm call. I like to think I had some role in that transformation. Yet I still hear heartbreaking stories from women who are large animal practitioners—stories of frustration about being paid less than men, lack of accommodation for pregnancies and family, skepticism from dairymen and even other veterinarians. There is a persistent gender pay gap in the profession. We still have a way to go for women to be treated as equals, but I hope my story illustrating that women who show up and demonstrate they can do the job can, ultimately, effect positive change.

Of course, my story didn't end with me in the barn for the rest of my career. My path took me first to California and then back east and on to graduate school. I earned my PhD in reproductive physiology and embarked on a career in research, helping to develop new medicines for a variety of species—a different way of helping animals and veterinarians. At every step, the lessons I learned while practicing in Utah, with all those beautiful cows, built the foundation of my professional journey. Show up no matter the weather, don't let them see how scared you are, work your heart out, pay no attention to folks who think you don't belong, and do your best. Above all, believe in yourself—and don't mind getting dirty.

Acknowledgments

THIS STORY IS AS TRUE as I could make it, given that my memory is not perfect. I have changed the names of some of the key characters, while others I have kept. Many of the dairymen in the story have since died, but I was able to track down Greg Mauchley and Crae Fuhriman, who gave their permission to use their names and photos. Thanks to the relatives of the Mickelsons, who remembered the lady cow vet and shared old stories. They reminded me that the cow pictured in the hay on the cover was named Pinky. Without the support and encouragement of the Utah and Idaho dairymen, I never would have had the opportunity to practice. Thanks to the LDS community of Logan for their understanding, acceptance, and support when I most needed it.

Several writing teachers helped me bring my memories to life, and their insights and encouragement made this a better book. I thank Alexandra Soiseth for her patience in working through multiple drafts, and Marcia Bradley who saw the core of the story, and was incredibly encouraging. I am so grateful for their support. I also thank Susan Aiello, a friend, fellow veterinarian and talented editor, for encouragement and editing several drafts of the manuscript.

And finally, thanks to my parents, Josie and Dusty Rhodes, for bringing me up to believe that a girl could do anything she set her mind to, and for creating a home where logical thinking, taking risks, and challenging the status quo were considered virtues.

About the Author

LINDA RHODES began her career as a dairy cow veterinarian after she graduated from the University of Pennsylvania *summa cum laude* in 1978. After several years in dairy practice, she was granted a fellowship at Cornell University, where she obtained her PhD in 1988. The rest of her career was spent in the pharmaceutical industry, helping to develop medicines for many species of animals. She retired in 2016 and has subsequently served on several corporate and start-up boards in the animal health industry. She has received the Iron Paw Award for her lifetime achievements. *Breaking the Barnyard Barrier* is her first book.